T0296420

# FAST FACTS FOR DEMENTIA CARE

**Carol A. Miller, MSN, RN-BC**, is a Clinical Instructor, Frances Payne Bolton School of Nursing, and a Clinical Nurse Specialist, Care and Counseling, Private Geriatric Care Practice. She is the author of *Nursing for Wellness in Older Adults*, now in its sixth edition, which received an *American Journal of Nursing* Book of the Year Award in Gerontology, and *Nurse's Toolbook for Promoting Wellness*. Ms. Miller has published more than 100 nursing articles and textbook chapters. She has taught at Cleveland State University and The University of Akron, among other institutions. She has served as a spokesperson for a national health education campaign on issues related to caregiving, a role that involved appearances on hundreds of radio and TV programs, including *Good Morning America*.

Ms. Miller has served on the professional advisory board of the Alzheimer's Association and is widely recognized as an expert in the care of older adults. Her expertise in person-centered care for people with dementia comes from over three decades of clinical practice, research, and writing. Clinical settings include a geropsychiatric program, inpatient and outpatient hospital programs, long-term care settings, and home and community settings. Since 1990, she has addressed the needs of people with dementia and their care partners in many settings as a consultant, advisor, and direct care provider through her geriatric care management practice.

# FAST FACTS FOR DEMENTIA CARE

## What Nurses Need to Know in a Nutshell

Carol A. Miller, MSN, RN-BC

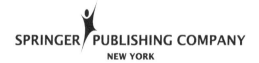

SPRINGER PUBLISHING COMPANY
NEW YORK

Springer Publishing Company, LLC
11 West 42nd Street
New York, NY 10036
www.springerpub.com

Acquisitions Editor: Margaret Zuccarini
Composition: S4Carlisle Publishing Services

ISBN: 978-0-8261-2036-6
E-book ISBN: 978-0-8261-2037-3

12 13 14/ 5 4 3 2 1

The author and the publisher of this Work have made every effort to use sources believed to be reliable to provide information that is accurate and compatible with the standards generally accepted at the time of publication. Because medical science is continually advancing, our knowledge base continues to expand. Therefore, as new information becomes available, changes in procedures become necessary. We recommend that the reader always consult current research and specific institutional policies before performing any clinical procedure. The author and publisher shall not be liable for any special, consequential, or exemplary damages resulting, in whole or in part, from the readers' use of, or reliance on, the information contained in this book. The publisher has no responsibility for the persistence or accuracy of URLs for external or third-party Internet Web sites referred to in this publication and does not guarantee that any content on such Web sites is, or will remain, accurate or appropriate.

Library of Congress Cataloging-in-Publication Data

Miller, Carol A.
  Fast facts for dementia care : what nurses need to know in a nutshell/Carol A. Miller.
     p. ; cm.
  Includes bibliographical references.
  ISBN-13: 978-0-8261-2036-6
  ISBN-10: 0-8261-2036-9
  ISBN-13: 978-0-8261-2037-3 (e-book)
  I. Title.
    [DNLM: 1.  Dementia—nursing.  2.  Geriatric Nursing—methods.  WY 152]
  LC classification not assigned
  616.8'3—dc23

                                                                              2012004635

Printed in the United States of America by Hamilton Printing

# Contents

# Preface

If you are a nurse working in an adult health setting, you most likely care for patients whose mental status is altered during all or some of the time you provide care. It's also likely that many of your patients who are older than 75 or 80 years have a diagnosis of dementia and others have manifestations of dementia, but have not been "officially labeled" as such. In addition, if you work in an acute care setting, it's likely that many of your patients at any age experience an altered mental status due to delirium during the course of care. Despite the increasing awareness of delirium as a cause of altered mental status, many of these patients will not be diagnosed as such. In all these circumstances, one of your primary nursing responsibilities is to address the needs of patients whose mental status is compromised, whether it is due to dementia, delirium, or a combination of these conditions.

*Fast Facts for Dementia Care* has evolved out of more than three decades of my gerontological nursing experiences caring for people with dementia in a wide range of clinical settings, including acute care, long-term care, and home and community settings. Its intent is to help you incorporate a person-centered approach in your usual nursing care as you address the unique needs of people who have dementia. The basic premise is that although the short-term nature of the care setting focuses on nursing interventions for the immediate medical problems, nurses have numerous opportunities to incorporate dementia-specific interventions in care plans. This approach does not require extra time; in many circumstances, it saves time because it prevents problems from occurring or addresses issues before they escalate. These person-centered interventions for dementia can have a significant positive effect on the care you provide. In addition, if you are familiar with the dementia-related issues and resources discussed in this book, you have numerous opportunities to suggest referrals for longer-term follow-up.

Chapters in Part I discuss types of dementia and other commonly occurring conditions that have similar manifestations; these chapters focus on nursing responsibilities for assessment and management of patients who have dementia. Chapters in Part II describe the application of a person-centered approach to address issues that are commonly associated with different stages of dementia. Part III discusses issues that nurses address in specific care settings and focuses on nursing interventions for pain, safety, and communication. The chapters in Part IV are a guide to addressing some of the behaviors commonly associated with dementia. The last two chapters address ethical and legal issues and nursing strategies to address caregiver needs. A major emphasis throughout the text is on relatively simple interventions that nurses can incorporate in their discharge plans to teach families and care partners about sources of information and support to address the needs of people with dementia.

Although some terminology in this book may seem cumbersome or unfamiliar, I have made every effort to use terms that are consistent with my focus on person-centered care. For example, I consistently use the phrase "person with dementia" to emphasize the personhood of the patient who has dementia as a chronic condition affecting his or her care. I also use the term "care partners" rather than "caregiver" to emphasize that people with dementia are not passive recipients of care, particularly during mild and even moderate stages. This phrase is appropriate because the care of people with dementia requires the *partnership* of many personal and professional support people working together to address this complex situation. The term "caregiver" is used in some chapters in reference to needs of family members and support people who are most directly affected, particularly when the person has moderate or severe dementia.

Many years ago, one of my clients told me, "I try to learn from my dementia so I can help others." This client is one of the hundreds of individuals with dementia who have enhanced my professional nursing education and research as I have developed my expertise in dementia. As a geriatric care manager, I have often advocated for my clients when they receive care in hospitals, emergency rooms, their homes, and long-term care settings. In all these settings, I have discussed their care with nurses who are experts in addressing medical issues, but have little or no knowledge base for addressing issues that arise out of their patients' dementia. In this book, I share the expertise I have developed so nurses in all settings can address the unique and challenging needs of their patients who are individuals with dementia. It is my hope that the information in this book will not only improve care for people with dementia, but also improve professional life for nurses who care for them.

*Carol A. Miller, MSN, RN-BC*

# Acknowledgments

First and foremost, I appreciate the many people with dementia and their families and care partners whom I have cared for and care about as a nurse. I value the challenges they have presented and the opportunities I have had for applying my expertise and learning from them. I am grateful for Pat Rehm's unending support and understanding as I have engaged in this writing venture, and I also appreciate my family cheerleaders who provide many expressions of encouragement.

# Dementia: What It Is, What It Is Not, and What Nurses Can Do

# Defining Dementia

## INTRODUCTION

*Some changes in cognition occur in even the healthiest older adults, but any changes that significantly interfere with usual functioning and quality of life are associated with pathologic conditions. Although our understanding of cognitive function has increased considerably in recent decades, cognitive changes remain one of the most complex and challenging aspects of geriatric care. Nurses who provide care for older adults in any care setting need to be knowledgeable about cognitive changes so they can accurately assess and address this important aspect of functioning and quality of life. This chapter, which presents basic information about normal cognitive aging and dementia, lays the groundwork for incorporating a person-centered approach when you care for older adults who are cognitively compromised.*

In this chapter, you will learn:

1. Normal cognitive aging
2. Strategies to facilitate health teaching in older adults
3. The definition and types of dementia
4. How dementia is diagnosed

5. Stages of dementia
6. Nursing responsibilities related to identification of dementia

## NORMAL COGNITIVE AGING

Some cognitive changes are an inherent part of aging; however, these changes do not progress to the point that they significantly affect functioning, personality, or behavior. In fact, some aspects of cognition improve as we age. In the absence of pathologic brain changes, healthy older adults experience the following changes in cognition by the time they are in their 70s or 80s:

• Better skills: wisdom, creativity, common sense, coordination of facts and ideas, and breadth of knowledge and experience
• Diminished skills: abstraction, calculation, word fluency, verbal comprehension, spatial orientation, and inductive reasoning
• Memory for details of events of the past may decrease, but short-term memory should not decline
• Difficulty finding the right word quickly
• Slower processing of information

Nurses can differentiate between normal and pathologic cognitive changes by assessing the degree to which the changes affect functioning.

*FAST FACTS in a NUTSHELL*

If cognitive changes noticeably limit the person's functioning, it is likely that dementia or some other pathologic process is the underlying cause.

🌀 CLINICAL SNAPSHOT: Normal cognitive aging may cause older adults to have momentary difficulty remembering where they left their car, but if older adults have dementia they may not remember that they drove a car.

It is important to remember that conditions such as depression, medication effects, vision or hearing impairment, and physical or emotional stress can affect cognitive function in people of any age. Older adults, however, are more likely than their younger counterparts to have one or more of the conditions that have a negative impact on cognitive functioning. Thus, older adults are likely to have difficulty processing information and this limitation can affect the health teaching that is integral to comprehensive nursing care. Table 1.1 describes strategies that nurses can use to facilitate health teaching for older adults.

**TABLE 1.1 Nursing Strategies to Facilitate Health Teaching**

| Condition | Nursing Implications for Health Teaching |
|---|---|
| Age-related cognitive changes | Allow more time for information processing; use simple written and visual materials; provide small amounts of information at one time; reinforce information with repetition; and make the information relevant to the person's experiences. |
| Impaired vision | Use large type and good contrast letters and pictures; provide adequate non-glare lighting; if the person wears eyeglasses, make sure the glasses are accessible and clean. |
| Impaired hearing | Pace your speech appropriately; use amplifier device if needed; position yourself face-to-face with the patient; articulate words, but do not exaggerate; do not chew gum; reduce background noise as much as possible; if the person uses a hearing aid, make sure it is available and functional. |
| Physical stress | Ensure as much comfort as possible by addressing pain, thirst, hunger, discomfort, fatigue, and other conditions as much as possible. |
| Medications | Assess and address medication effects that may interfere with cognitive function (e.g., the anticholinergic effects of many medications can compromise mental status). |

*(continued)*

---

**TABLE 1.1  Nursing Strategies to Facilitate Health Teaching  (continued)**

| Condition | Nursing Implications for Health Teaching |
| --- | --- |
| Emotional stress | Encourage patients to express feelings; use good listening skills; be fully present to patients; teach simple breathing exercises for stress reduction; encourage the presence of supportive friends/family. |

---

================*FAST FACTS in a NUTSHELL*

Nurses can facilitate health teaching by using strategies that address both cognitive changes and many of the factors that interfere with optimal cognitive function (Table 1.1).

## DEFINITION AND TYPES OF DEMENTIA

The term *dementia* refers to a group of chronic pathologic conditions characterized by a progressive decline in cognitive abilities. Dementia typically begins with a gradual onset of cognitive changes that are difficult to distinguish from normal aging; these changes are sometimes called mild cognitive impairment or MCI. As dementia progresses, it eventually affects behavior, personality, and all aspects of functioning and is considered a terminal condition. There is no single test for dementia and even the most skilled geriatric practitioners find it challenging to diagnose dementia in its earliest stages.

Alzheimer's disease, which was first described in medical literature in 1907, is the most common and widely recognized type of dementia. Alzheimer's disease is characterized by hallmark pathologic changes that affect specific regions of the brain. A second distinct type of dementia, called vascular or multi-infarct dementia, was identified in the 1970s when scientists documented vascular changes in autopsied brains. This type is caused by a major stroke or by the cumulative effects of many minor strokes. When vascular dementia is caused by a major stroke it has an acute onset, does not always progress, and may even improve with treatment. This type, therefore, may not fit the characteristics of gradual, progressive, and irreversible. It is important to recognize, however, that "pure" vascular dementia is rare because most people with vascular brain changes also have a significant degree of the pathologic changes of Alzheimer's disease (Sabbagh, McCarthy, & Martin, 2011). When people exhibit characteristics of both vascular dementia and Alzheimer's disease, the term "mixed dementia" is used.

In recent decades, the increasing use of longitudinal studies and more complex brain imaging techniques has enabled scientists to describe many other types of dementia, such as Lewy body dementia and frontotemporal dementia. Table 1.2 outlines distinguishing features of these four most commonly diagnosed types. Causes of dementia that occur less commonly include head trauma, Parkinson's disease, multiple sclerosis, Huntington's disease, Creutzfeldt-Jakob disease, normal

### TABLE 1.2 Distinguishing Features of Four Major Types of Dementia

| Type | Distinguishing Features |
| --- | --- |
| Alzheimer's disease | Slow onset typically beginning during the seventh decade but may begin earlier; steady progression over 10 or more years; loss of short-term memory is a prominent characteristic during all stages; gradually affects personality, behavior, and all aspects of functioning |
| Vascular dementia | Gradual onset due to cumulative effects of small strokes OR sudden onset if related to a major stroke; risk factors include strokes, heart disease, high blood pressure, and atrial fibrillation; irregular course or possible improvement depending on causative factors and presence of other brain pathologies |

*(continued)*

8 PART I DEMENTIA: WHAT NURSES CAN DO

**TABLE 1.2 Distinguishing Features of Four Major Types of Dementia (continued)**

| Type | Distinguishing Features |
| --- | --- |
| Lewy body dementia | Often misdiagnosed as Alzheimer's, especially during early stages; slow onset with progressive decline in cognitive, behavioral, and motor symptoms; significant fluctuations in functioning, particularly when the person is medically unstable; highly sensitive to neuroleptic medications |
| Frontotemporal dementia | Often begins during the sixth or seventh decade with personality and behavioral changes; initially affects language, social skills, thought processing, and decision-making skills; memory impairments occur later |

pressure hydrocephalus (NPH), and AIDS. These causes often impair some aspect of physical functioning before affecting cognition, whereas changes in cognition, behavior, and personality are generally the initial manifestations of Alzheimer's, vascular, Lewy body, or frontotemporal dementia.

## DIAGNOSIS OF DEMENTIA

Dementia is both a retrospective and a "rule-out" diagnosis: It is retrospective because, with the exception of stroke-associated dementia, the manifestations develop over many years; it is a rule-out process because the initial workup is directed toward identifying any treatable condition that can cause similar cognitive, behavioral, and personality changes. A diagnostic evaluation for dementia generally includes all the following: a comprehensive history of changes in cognition, personality, and behavior; a complete physical evaluation to identify any causative medical conditions; a functional assessment; and a neuropsychological evaluation. This evaluation is very complex and involves clinical examinations as well as blood tests and imaging tests of the brain.

Even today with advanced imaging techniques and knowledge about clinical manifestations of different types of dementia, it is difficult to diagnose dementia during its earliest stages. As the cognitive changes progress and dementia begins to affect other aspects of functioning—such as personality, behavior, and physical functioning—it is easier to differentiate among the types of dementia. Another complicating factor is that an individual may have pathologic changes of two or more types of dementia at the same time, particularly with Alzheimer's and vascular dementia.

In 2011, the National Institute on Aging and the Alzheimer's Association issued a major report on criteria for diagnosis of dementia based on the past 27 years of research and experience. Exhibit 1.1 summarizes the pertinent clinical criteria for all-cause dementia that these groups developed.

**Exhibit 1.1  Core Clinical Criteria for Diagnosis of Dementia**

Presence of cognitive or behavioral symptoms that:

- Interfere with ability to function in usual activities
- Represent a decline in level of functioning
- Are not due to delirium or a psychiatric disorder

Cognitive impairment is assessed through a combination of:

- History-taking from the patient and a knowledgeable informant
- Mental status examination or neuropsychological testing

*(continued)*

**Exhibit 1.1**    *(continued)*

Cognitive or behavioral impairment in two or more of the following aspects of functioning:

- Impaired ability to acquire and remember new information (e.g., repetitive questions)
- Impaired reasoning, judgment, or handling of complex tasks (e.g., poor understanding of safety risks)
- Impaired visuospatial abilities (e.g., inability to recognize common objects)
- Impaired language function (e.g., significant word-finding impairment)
- Changes in personality or behavior (e.g., apathy, mood fluctuations, or socially inappropriate actions)

*Source:* Adapted from McKhann et al. (2011) with permission from Elsevier.

A major clinical implication of an accurate diagnosis of dementia is that all treatable causes are identified as early as possible so that they can be addressed. Another clinical implication is that nurses need to know how different types of dementia can affect functioning. For example, patients with Lewy body dementia may have an increased sensitivity to medications that affect the central nervous system, so nurses need to be cautious about doses of those medications. Another example is that patients with frontotemporal dementia may retain memory skills but manifest significant personality changes or impairment in social skills.

*FAST FACTS in a NUTSHELL*

Dementia is a very complex diagnosis that requires comprehensive evaluations of all aspects of functioning and an overview of changes over time (Exhibit 1.1).

## STAGES OF DEMENTIA

Although specific characteristics are associated with each type of dementia, many characteristics are common to all types of dementia. Common characteristics of mild, moderate, and advanced stages of dementia are as follows:

*Mild Dementia*
- Cognitive impairments that interfere with the performance of familiar tasks
- Impaired judgment, problemsolving, and decision-making skills
- Difficulty processing visual or spatial information
- Significant problems with speaking or writing
- Withdrawal from usual work or social activities
- Changes in mood or personality (e.g., increased anxiety, irritability, depression)

*Moderate Dementia*
- Continued decline in all aspects of cognition
- Increasing confusion
- Need for some assistance or direction with usual activities
- Disorientation to time or place
- Frequent or intermittent occurrence of neuropsychological manifestations (e.g., delusions, hallucinations, agitation, depression, apathy)

## Advanced Dementia

- Major impairments in all aspects of cognition
- Inability to recognize familiar people or surroundings
- Need for assistance in all activities of daily living
- Disrupted sleep/wake cycle
- Significant personality changes and behavioral manifestations (e.g., agitation, repetitive behaviors, delusions, hallucinations)
- Diminished physical functioning, including incontinence and impaired mobility

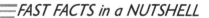

## FAST FACTS in a NUTSHELL

Dementia progresses through mild, moderate, and advanced stages and each stage is characterized by progressive changes in cognition, behavior, and functioning.

Because dementia is a progressive condition, these characteristics change and are often described according to clinical rating scales. Rating scales are typically based on characteristics of Alzheimer's disease, so they may not be applicable to other types of dementia, nor do they account for the many conditions that occur concomitantly with dementia and cause fluctuations in functioning and cognition. In addition, dementia affects people in individualized ways, and people with dementia do not fit neatly into categories. Nurses can find detailed information about rating scales at the Internet sites listed in the Resources in a Nutshell section at the end of this chapter.

It is important to note that stages of dementia describe the progression of the condition and its effects on the person's functioning and are not related in any way to the person's age. The typical age for onset of dementia is during the seventh decade or later, but dementia can occur in people in their 40s or 50s. When dementia occurs before the age of 60, it is called early-onset disease.

## NURSING RESPONSIBILITIES RELATED TO IDENTIFICATION OF DEMENTIA

Nurses in most health care settings are not responsible for diagnosing dementia or using dementia rating scales, but nurses are responsible in all settings for assessing changes in mental status during the course of usual nursing care. Every clinical setting has mental status assessment forms that generally include criteria such as orientation, alertness, and contact with reality (e.g., hallucinations). In addition, some clinical settings use standardized mental status assessment forms, such as the mini-mental status examination with a total score of 30 points. No matter what assessment format is used, additional assessment skills are necessary because the assessment tools do not identify underlying conditions that affect mental status.

It also is imperative to identify concomitant conditions in people who already have dementia and avoid attributing a change in functioning as "simply" a progression of dementia. It is important to be on the alert for treatable components whenever the person with dementia experiences a change in functioning. For example, an infection or electrolyte imbalance can affect overall functioning and mental status in older adults, and nurses are in a key position to assess for these conditions and take appropriate action rather than attributing the changes to dementia. Chapters 2 and 3 discuss many of the conditions that affect people with dementia or are mistakenly attributed to dementia.

━━━━━━━━━━━━━━━━*FAST FACTS in a NUTSHELL*

In addition to using standard mental status assessment forms, assess for conditions that affect cognitive function, especially those that can be addressed through nursing interventions.

✹ **CLINICAL SNAPSHOT:** Nurses can assess and address the conditions listed in Table 1.1 that can compromise cognitive function and interfere with health teaching.

✹ **CLINICAL SNAPSHOT: THROUGH THE STAGES OF DEMENTIA**

Mild Dementia

During the past few years Sophie D, a 73-year-old widow living alone, has become more and more forgetful about keeping appointments. In contrast to her usual meticulous style of dressing, she wears soiled and mismatched clothes and no longer goes to the beauty shop. She has difficulty shopping for groceries and now walks to the nearby fast food stores for most of her meals. The family has noticed that she no longer sends birthday cards to grandchildren as she has faithfully done for many years. She has little awareness of these changes and, in fact, is quite defensive when anyone questions her about memory problems.

Moderate Dementia

Sophie is now 76 years old and has recently moved to an assisted living facility because she was no longer safe at home. Staff members provide direction or assistance for all

(continued)

activities of daily living, including giving her medications, setting out her clothing every morning, and reminding her about using the toilet every few hours. She attends group activities a couple times a day and especially enjoys the music events. She frequently asks about when her family will visit but does not remember that she had visitors an hour ago. She spends much of her time looking for misplaced objects and sometimes takes things belonging to other residents and believes they are her own.

### Advanced Dementia

Sophie is 81 years old and has moved to a nursing facility because she needs full assistance with all activities of daily living. She has lost weight and complains about the mechanical soft diet that is prescribed because of her difficulty with chewing and swallowing. When her family visits, she usually does not recognize them but she says they are "very nice people." All cognitive skills are significantly impaired and it is difficult to carry on a normal conversation. She has no memory for recent or remote events and often asks where her husband is, despite the fact that he has been dead for 16 years. She has difficulty walking and has fallen a couple times because she does not call for help when she needs to get out of bed.

# *RESOURCES in a NUTSHELL*

*Alzheimer's Association*
*www.alz.org*
- Alzheimer's disease, including local resources for professionals and caregivers

*(continued)*

(*continued*)

### American Medical Association

*www.ama-assn.org/ama1/pub/upload/mm/433/aging_vs_dementia.pdf*

- Differentiating normal aging and dementia

### Hartford Institute for Geriatric Nursing

*consultgerirn.org*

- Normal cognitive aging
- Assessing cognitive function
- Mental status assessment
- Best practices in nursing care to older adults with dementia

### Helpguide

*www.helpguide.org*

- Information about memory loss and aging

### Lewy Body Dementia Association

*www.lbda.org*

- Information and resources about Lewy body dementia

### National Institute on Aging

*www.nia.nih.gov/Alzheimers*

- Research and information about Alzheimer's disease

### National Institutes of Neurological Disorders and Stroke

*www.ninds.nih.gov/disorders*

- Overview of types of dementia

# 2

# Distinguishing Between Dementia and Delirium

## INTRODUCTION

*Although delirium has been documented in patients for centuries, in recent years it has been addressed as a commonly occurring condition that is serious, preventable, treatable, and often unrecognized. In addition, it can have serious consequences—including death—when it is not recognized and addressed. Older adults with dementia have the double disadvantage of having a higher incidence of delirium and having it overlooked as a separate and treatable condition.*

In this chapter, you will learn:

1. Characteristics of delirium in people with dementia
2. How to assess for delirium and delirium plus dementia
3. Nursing actions to address delirium

## WHAT IS DELIRIUM?

*Delirium* is a medical syndrome characterized by:

- Abrupt change in mental status
- Abnormal level of consciousness
- Fluctuations in mental status
- Disturbances in thought, memory, attention, behavior, perception, and orientation
- Evidence of concomitant physiologic condition

Types of delirium are hypoactive (lethargic, stuporous), hyperactive (agitated, restless), and mixed (fluctuating between hypoactive and hyperactive). It is difficult to recognize hypoactive delirium because it is not consistent with the usual perception of delirium as a hyperactive state.

Delirium is associated with serious consequences, including:

- Longer hospital stays
- Increased death rate
- Increased dependency and functional impairment
- Increased risk of long-term cognitive impairment
- Exacerbation of dementia
- Higher use of indwelling catheters
- Higher use of physical restraints
- Higher rates of permanent residency in long-term care facilities

═══════════════════*FAST FACTS in a NUTSHELL*

People with dementia have a double disadvantage: They are more likely to develop delirium and more likely to have serious consequences.

## WHAT ARE THE RISK FACTORS ASSOCIATED WITH DELIRIUM?

In addition to dementia being a risk factor for delirium, the following conditions can increase the risk:

- Increased age
- Pain
- Infections
- Surgery (especially cardiac or orthopedic)
- Medications (especially those with high anticholinergic properties)
- Physiologic disturbances (e.g., hypoxia, dehydration, electrolyte imbalance)
- Pathologic conditions (e.g., stroke, metabolic disorders)
- Sleep deprivation

Usually several interacting conditions contribute to the on-set of delirium, so it is important to assess for more than one causative factor.

Dementia increases the risk for delirium and it also increases the risk that delirium will not be recognized and treated. Because dementia inherently involves altered cognitive function and an unpredictable course, signs of delirium may be falsely attributed to the underlying dementia. Thus, it is imperative to know the person's usual level of cognitive function and to observe for even subtle changes that may be associated with treatable conditions. Nurses need to ask family members and care partners about the person's usual level of functioning and document this information so changes can be identified.

=============================*FAST FACTS in a NUTSHELL*

Whenever changes in mental status are observed in people with dementia, check for signs of delirium.

## HOW TO RECOGNIZE DELIRIUM PLUS DEMENTIA

Because impaired cognitive function is an inherent characteristic of both dementia and delirium, it is difficult to distinguish between these two conditions. Table 2.1 summarizes distinguishing features of dementia and delirium.

The Confusion Assessment Method (Inouye et al., 1990) is widely recognized as an easy-to-use standardized tool to identify delirium (Figure 2.1). Additional resources related to the Confusion Assessment Method, including models for people with dementia and in intensive care units, are listed in the Resources in a Nutshell at the end of this chapter.

## HOW TO RECOGNIZE AND ADDRESS CAUSES OF DELIRIUM

Onset or progression of physiologic disorders can precipitate delirium, and this may be more difficult to detect in people with dementia who cannot communicate accurately about their symptoms. Thus, it is important to obtain objective

**TABLE 2.1  Distinguishing Features of Dementia and Delirium**

| Characteristic | Dementia | Delirium |
| --- | --- | --- |
| Onset | Gradual | Sudden |
| Development | Slowly progressive over years | Rapid changes over hours |
| Attention | Can focus on task | Noticeably impaired, easily distracted |
| Consciousness | Alert and stable | Impaired and fluctuating |
| Speech | Confused but consistent | Incoherent |
| Course | Progressive, irreversible | Reversible if all causes are treated |

**CONFUSION ASSESSMENT METHOD (CAM)**

Features 1 and 2 plus 3 OR 4 indicates delirium

1. ACUTE ONSET AND                                     2. INATTENTION
   FLUCTUATING COURSE
                                       AND
   Change from baseline                                Difficulty focusing
   Fluctuating behaviors                               Easily distracted


        AND        3. DISORGANIZED THINKING

                      Rambling or irrelevant conversation
                      Unclear or illogical flow
                      Unpredictable change of topics


                              OR


            4. ALTERED LEVEL OF CONSCIOUSNESS

               Hyperalert, lethargic, stupor, or coma

**FIGURE 2.1**    Confusion Assessment Method (CAM) for diagnosing delirium.

information as well as reported information from the person with dementia and that person's care partners. The following sections describe nursing actions to detect delirium in people with dementia. Figure 2.2 illustrates a flow chart for nursing assessment and interventions related to delirium. In addition, Chapter 10 addresses pain in people with dementia, which is a common cause of delirium.

## Infections

Infections—including pneumonia, dental abscesses, and urinary tract infections—are the most common causes of delirium. Identification of infection in people with dementia is not straightforward for the following reasons: (a) they

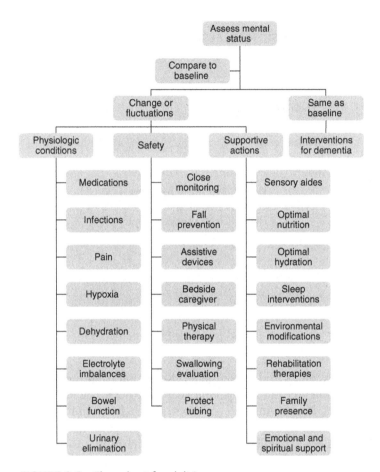

**FIGURE 2.2**  Flow chart for delirium.

may not be able to accurately report their symptoms; (b) if their baseline temperature is low, which is common among older adults, their temperature may register as normal but be elevated above their usual; and (c) older adults may have a delayed or absent temperature elevation when they have an infection.

Some nursing actions to detect infections include the following:

- Assess for pain, discomfort, and other physical changes
- Check temperature for an increase above the baseline
- Check urine specimen for indicators of urinary tract infection
- Note any changes in urinary elimination (e.g., incontinence, frequency, or urgency)
- Assess skin, joints, and oral cavity for inflammation or recent onset of abnormalities
- Assess respirations and lung sounds
- Observe for changes in mobility or any aspect of functioning
- Obtain orders for blood tests, sputum cultures, and chest x-rays as appropriate

═══════════════════════════════*FAST FACTS in a NUTSHELL*

What is the rationale for obtaining a urinalysis when a change in a patient's behavior is noted? Rationale: A urinary tract infection is a common cause of delirium in older adults.

## Physiologic Alterations

In addition to infections, other physiologic alterations that cause delirium include hypoxia, dehydration, malnutrition, fecal impactions, hypo- or hyperglycemia, and electrolyte imbalances. The following nursing actions assess for physiologic alterations:

- Assess all vital signs
- Check pulse oximetry
- Check blood glucose with glucometer
- Review lab work, including electrolytes and blood counts, and obtain orders for appropriate tests
- Monitor intake and output

- Assess nutritional status
- Check bowel sounds
- Obtain information about recent bowel movements
- Perform digital rectal exam for fecal impaction
- Assess skin, oral mucous membrane, and urine specific gravity for indications of dehydration

## ═══════════════════════FAST FACTS in a NUTSHELL

Take a detective-like approach to identify conditions that may be causing delirium.

🌀 CLINICAL SNAPSHOT: Mr. M lives with his wife, who reported that the police brought him home after he had gone outside during the night in his pajamas. When the visiting nurse assessed him, she could find no signs of infection, but Mrs. M reported that a crown had fallen off one of her husband's teeth. Based on the nurse's advice, Mrs. M took her husband to his dentist, who found that he had an abscessed tooth. After the dental issue resolved, Mr. M had no further episodes of leaving the house at night.

## Medications

Medications, particularly those with strong anticholinergic properties, are a very common cause of delirium (Table 2.2). Indirect effects of medications also can cause delirium (e.g., diuretic-induced dehydration or electrolyte imbalance). Although most nurses do not prescribe medications, all nurses are responsible for assessing for altered mental status as an adverse effect. Nursing guidelines related to medications as a cause of delirium include:

- Be on the alert for drug interactions and recognize that any physiologic substance—including food, fluids,

### TABLE 2.2 Medications That Can Cause Delirium

| Type | Example |
|---|---|
| Pre-anesthesia drugs | atropine (Atropen), scopolamine (Hyoscine) |
| Bladder antispasmodics | oxybutynin (Ditropan) |
| Antihistamines | chlorpheniramine (Chlor-Trimeton), diphenhydramine (Benadryl) |
| Antianxiety agents | benzodiazepines (e.g., Valium, Xanax) |
| Antipsychotics | chlorpromazine (Thorazine), fluphenazine (Prolixin) |
| Antidepressants | amitriptyline (Elavil), imipramine (Tofranil) |
| Movement disorders | benztropine (Cogentin), trihexphenidyl (Artane) |
| Cardiovascular drugs | disopyramide (Norpace), digitalis (Digoxin), propanolol (Inderal) |
| Motion sickness, nausea | meclizine (Antivert), promethazine (Phenergan) |
| Muscle spasm | methocarbamol (Robaxin) |
| Analgesics, especially narcotics | meperidine (Demerol) |
| Gastrointestinal agents | dicyclomine (Bentyl), cimetidine (Tagamet) |

herbs, vitamins, alcohol, nicotine, and nonprescription medications—can alter medications.
- Check for recent changes in medication regimen but recognize that some drugs that have been taken for a long time can cause delirium at any time, especially in conjunction with other physiologic alterations.
- Recognize that older adults are more susceptible to medication-induced delirium because of age-related changes in the brain.
- Recognize that a change in mental status can be caused by withdrawal from prescribed medications, illegal drugs, or alcohol.
- Obtain serum levels of medications that should be monitored.
- Avoid using medications for addressing behavioral issues that can be resolved with non-pharmacologic interventions.

===*FAST FACTS in a NUTSHELL*

Combined effects of several anticholinergic medications can cause delirium.

**CLINICAL SNAPSHOT:** Mrs. N was brought to the emergency room for evaluation of recent-onset confusion. She has been taking oxybutynin (Ditropan) for overactive bladder and recently started taking Tylenol PM (acetaminophen and diphenhydramine/Benadryl) at bedtime and again during the night for difficulty sleeping due to arthritis pain. The geriatrician discontinued the oxybutynin and prescribed darifenacin (Enablex) and instructed Mrs. N to take plain acetaminophen at bedtime. Mrs. N's mental status returned to normal within a couple days.

## HOW TO ADDRESS THE NEEDS OF PEOPLE WITH DEMENTIA AND DELIRIUM

### Safety

Delirium in people with dementia is associated with significant personal safety risks, such as falls and aspiration pneumonia. These risks are magnified if the person is unable to recognize the need for help or unable to use call lights or other devices to obtain help in a timely manner. Delirium also increases the risk for the patient removing tubes connected with medically important, even life-sustaining, devices. The following nursing actions promote safety for people with dementia:

- Position patient close to the nursing station and monitor frequently
- Arrange for bedside caregiver or family attendant to observe behaviors, prevent injuries, protect medical tubing,

and provide cognitive and emotional support (e.g., orientation, reassurance, information)
- Obtain physical therapy evaluation and follow recommendations related to mobility assistance and use of assistive devices
- Avoid the use of physical restraints and follow institutional policies for fall prevention
- Use soft items or mittens to prevent the patient from pulling tubes out
- Obtain swallowing evaluation and follow speech therapist's guidelines for safe eating and drinking techniques (e.g., thickened liquids, use of straws)

===== *FAST FACTS in a NUTSHELL*

Interventions for safety must be individualized and address the changes associated with both dementia and delirium.

🔹 **CLINICAL SNAPSHOT:** Mr. F uses a walker for safe mobility, but when he is in the hospital with delirium, he forgets to call for help and will get out of bed if he sees his walker. Nursing staff keep the walker out of sight because he does remember to call for help to find his walker.

## Comfort and Physical Needs

Nurses need to be proactive in addressing physical needs because dementia and delirium compromise one's ability to ask for assistance. In addition, nurses provide supportive interventions to address the emotional and spiritual needs of persons with dementia and their care partners. Nursing actions to address these needs include the following:

- Assess and address pain (see Chapter 10)
- Obtain dietary consultations to address nutritional and hydration issues

- Provide appropriate amounts of preferred foods and beverages and ensure that these are readily accessible
- Provide good oral and skin care
- Ensure access to sensory aids (e.g., clean eyeglasses, hearing devices)
- Limit noise as much as possible, but provide soothing music
- Provide orientation reminders (clocks, calendars, up-to-date information on dry-erase boards)
- Obtain physical therapy for safe mobility and exercise program
- Obtain occupational therapy for safety and independence in activities of daily living
- Promote optimal urinary elimination (frequent assistance, timely response to requests for help, avoid the use of indwelling catheters)
- Promote optimal bowel elimination (measures to prevent or address constipation or diarrhea)
- Promote sleep (comfort measures, avoid sedatives/hypnotics)
- Obtain dental consultation to address issues with teeth, dentures, or oral cavity
- Provide emotional support (listening, presence, encourage expression of feelings)
- Encourage presence of supportive care partners
- Address spiritual needs

## RESOURCES in a NUTSHELL

### Hartford Institute for Geriatric Nursing

*consultgerirn.org*
- The Confusion Assessment Method (CAM), *Try This*, Issue 13, and video illustrating application of the assessment tool

*(continued)*

*(continued)*

- The Confusion Assessment Method for the ICU (CAM-ICU), *Try This,* Issue 25
- Assessing and Managing Delirium in Older Adults with Dementia, *Try This,* Issue D8
- Working with Families of Hospitalized Older Adults with Dementia, *Try This,* Issue D10

# 3

## Identifying Conditions
## That Mimic Dementia

## INTRODUCTION

*Because dementia is a "rule-out" diagnosis, a goal of the diagnostic process is to identify other conditions that can cause changes in cognition. Even after an initial diagnosis, however, it is important to frequently assess for conditions that can cause mental changes because these are often overlooked in people with dementia. Nurses need to assess for not only the acute conditions that can cause cognitive changes as discussed in Chapter 2, but also for chronic medical conditions and medication effects that can mimic dementia. In addition, depression is a commonly occurring condition that is often misidentified as dementia.*

In this chapter, you will learn:

1. Medical conditions that can cause mental changes
2. Medication effects that can cause mental changes
3. Depression in older adults
4. Nursing assessment of conditions that mimic dementia
5. Nursing actions for conditions that mimic dementia

## MEDICAL CONDITIONS THAT CAN CAUSE MENTAL CHANGES

Undiagnosed medical conditions can cause cognitive changes and when these progress without being identified or treated, they can mimic dementia. Examples of conditions that develop slowly and have subtle manifestations include:

- Hypothyroidism
- Hyperthyroidism
- Anemia
- Vitamin $B_{12}$ deficiency
- Chronic infections (e.g., urinary tract infections)
- Repeated transient ischemic attacks (small vessel cerebrovascular disease)

## ═══════════════════════FAST FACTS in a NUTSHELL

Poorly controlled chronic conditions can cause or contribute to altered mental status.

**CLINICAL SNAPSHOT:** Mrs. G is being evaluated for memory problems which have worsened during the past 6 months. She has been taking levothyroxine (Synthroid) for many years, but you question whether she has been remembering to take it as prescribed and you ask when was the last time she had her hypothyroidism evaluated.

## MEDICATION EFFECTS THAT CAN CAUSE MENTAL CHANGES

Medications can cause mental changes in anyone, but older adults are at increased risk of having adverse effects and having these effects falsely attributed to dementia. When people with dementia experience additional cognitive changes, these

**TABLE 3.1 Adverse Medication Effects That Can Cause Mental Changes**

| Adverse Effect | Examples |
| --- | --- |
| Hyponatremia | Diuretics, antidepressants |
| Hypoglycemia | Diabetic medications, beta blockers |
| Hyperglycemia | Corticosteroids |
| Acidosis | Salicylates |
| Hormonal imbalances | Thyroid medications |
| Drug interactions | Anticholinergics |

changes may be falsely attributed to the dementia rather than to adverse medication effects. Cumulative effects of anticholinergic medications, as discussed in Chapter 2, are one of the most common causes of mental changes in older adults and people with dementia. In addition, drug interactions can potentiate the risk for mental changes, particularly when two or more drugs with anticholinergic action are taken. Table 3.1 lists other adverse medication effects that can cause mental changes, with examples of types of medications. Alcohol abuse is another common cause of mental changes that is often subtle or overlooked in older adults and people with dementia.

======*FAST FACTS in a NUTSHELL*

Cumulative effects of long-term medications can cause gradual mental changes that are mistaken for dementia.

**CLINICAL SNAPSHOT:** After Mrs. P, who had taken hydrochlorothiazide (Diuril) for many years, began taking citalopram (Celexa) for depression, she became increasingly confused. Her serum sodium level was 128 mEq/L, which was attributed to two medications that can cause hyponatremia. Her mental status returned to normal after the medications were changed.

## DEPRESSION IN OLDER ADULTS

Like delirium, depression is increasingly being addressed as a commonly occurring condition that is a serious and treatable cause of cognitive changes. Another similarity to delirium is that people with dementia have the double disadvantage of having a higher incidence of depression and having it overlooked as a separate and treatable condition. Although depression is not a normal part of aging, it occurs commonly in older adults due to the increased number of risk factors, such as:

• Cumulative or chronic stressors (e.g., losses, caregiver demands)
• Loss of social supports
• Medical conditions including stroke, dementia, cancer, myocardial infarction, and Parkinson's disease
• Functional limitations (especially recent onset)
• New medical diagnosis
• Chronic pain
• Alcohol or substance abuse

Consequences of depression include an increased risk for developing dementia, significantly diminished quality of life, and increased risk for committing suicide.

Dementia complicates the diagnosis of depression because the two conditions have overlapping manifestations, such as:

• Impaired memory
• Poor concentration
• Difficulty making decisions
• Withdrawal from social activity
• Apathy (i.e., lack of motivation and initiation)
• Irritability
• Personality changes

Despite the similarities, nurses can differentiate between these two conditions by considering the distinguishing characteristics of dementia and depression described in Table 3.2.

**TABLE 3.2 Distinguishing Features of Dementia and Depression**

| Characteristic | Dementia | Depression |
|---|---|---|
| Onset | Gradual, recognized by hindsight | Rapid, often associated with a triggering event |
| Awareness | Unaware or minimizes the symptoms | Exaggerated perception of cognitive deficits |
| Memory and attention | Impaired memory and attention but strong attempts to perform well | Cognitive deficits due to lack of motivation and inability to concentrate |
| Emotions | Affect changes easily in response to suggestions | Consistent feelings of sadness; tearfulness is common |
| Response to questions | Inaccurate but attempts to cover up deficits | Minimal response with little or no effort put forth |
| Decision making | Impaired due to difficulty processing information | Impaired due to lack of motivation |
| Personal appearance | Inappropriate dress due to impaired perceptions and thought processes | Little or no concern about appearance because of lack of motivation |
| Physical complaints | Inconsistent and vague complaints (e.g., tired, weak) | Sleep disturbances, gastrointestinal complaints, decreased energy |
| Social interaction | Enjoys social interaction and activities if they are not too challenging | Withdrawal from usual activities due to lack of enjoyment |
| Contact with reality | Misinterpretation of reality; if present, delusions are aimed at explaining deficits | Exaggerated sense of gloom and doom; auditory hallucinations or self-derogatory delusions |

================*FAST FACTS in a NUTSHELL*

Nurses can differentiate between dementia and depression by assessing a person's response to questions.

🌀 **CLINICAL SNAPSHOT:** When you ask Mr. D (who has early dementia) if he has noticed any changes in his memory, he replies, "I can tell you everything you'd ever want to know about the invasion of Normandy in World War II." When you ask Mrs. G (who is depressed) if she has noticed any changes in her memory, she replies, "I've been forgetting my appointments for lunch with friends, but that's OK because I've been staying in bed till afternoon."

## NURSING ASSESSMENT OF CONDITIONS THAT MIMIC DEMENTIA

A primary role of nurses is to take a detective-like approach to identifying conditions that can be mistakenly attributed to dementia. As discussed in Chapter 2, it is imperative to obtain information about the person's usual mental status so changes can be assessed and addressed. Whenever a change in mental status is assessed, nurses need to obtain the following information:

- Diagnostic measures that have been taken to identify medical conditions
- Changes in chronic conditions (e.g., poor control of diabetes, thyroid disorders, or congestive heart failure)
- Prescription and nonprescription medications being taken
- Recent changes in medications (new prescriptions and discontinuation of medications)

- Possible drug interactions, particularly with recently prescribed medications
- Use of alcohol or recreational substances (or withdrawal from these)

In addition to identifying physiologic conditions that affect mental status, nurses assess for depression. The American Geriatrics Society recommends periodic depression screening for all people beginning at age 60 and every 6 months for older persons with dementia. Many health care settings have easy-to-use depression screening tools, such as the Geriatric Depression Scale, which can be administered in 5 to 7 minutes. The Resources in a Nutshell section at the end of this chapter provides information about this and other screening tools. The U.S. Preventive Services Task Force (2009) recommends the following two questions to identify depression:

- During the past 2 weeks (or month) have you felt down, depressed, or hopeless?
- During the past 2 weeks (or month) have you felt little interest or pleasure in doing things?

An affirmative response to either of these questions indicates the need for further assessment with a formal depression scale.

## NURSING ACTIONS TO ADDRESS CONDITIONS THAT MIMIC DEMENTIA

Although nurses in short-term settings have limited opportunity to directly address conditions that mimic dementia, actions they can take include the following:

- Facilitate referrals for further evaluation immediately or after discharge

- Raise questions about adverse medication effects or drug interactions that can cause or contribute to mental changes
- Refer for social work assistance with plans for follow-up
- If specialized geriatric services are available within the institution (as discussed in Chapter 9), follow the procedure for a referral
- If there are indicators that the person is depressed, teach about the importance of having depression evaluated and refer to social worker for follow-up
- Teach persons with dementia and their care partners about reversible and treatable conditions that mimic dementia

*FAST FACTS in a NUTSHELL*

Be aware of opportunities to detect depression in people with dementia so you can initiate interventions.

🌀 **CLINICAL SNAPSHOT:** Mr. T, who has been admitted for exacerbation of congestive heart failure, expresses pervasive feelings of sadness and hopelessness. In addition, his wife reports that he has become more confused recently, even though he is on medications for dementia. After 3 days, his primary care practitioner says he is ready for discharge because his cardiac status is stable. You talk with Mr. and Mrs. T about depression and other conditions that can mimic dementia and you provide contact information for further evaluation with the comprehensive geriatric assessment program.

# RESOURCES in a NUTSHELL

*Stanford University*
*www.stanford.edu/~yesavage/GDS.html*
- Geriatric Depression Scale

*Hartford Institute for Geriatric Nursing*
*consultgerirn.org*
- The Geriatric Depression Scale, *Try This,* Issue 4, and video illustrating application of the assessment tool

*National Guideline Clearinghouse*
*www.guidelines.gov*
- Detection of depression in older adults with dementia

*Agency for Healthcare Research and Quality*
*www.ahrq.gov*
- Screening for depression

# 4

# Keeping Up to Date on Options
# for Management

## INTRODUCTION

*During the past two decades, two types of medications
have become the "gold standard" for treating people with
dementia, so nurses need to be aware of the guidelines
for these medications, even though they do not have primary responsibility for prescribing. In addition, nurses
often need to address questions about nonprescription
agents that are promoted for improving cognition not
only for people with dementia but also for all adults.*

In this chapter, you will learn:

1. Information about medications approved for treatment of dementia
2. How to teach about medications for dementia
3. How to address questions about nonprescription products
   promoted for dementia
4. Medications for management of dementia-related behaviors
5. Incorporating nonpharmacologic interventions for dementia into
   usual care

## MEDICATIONS APPROVED FOR TREATMENT OF DEMENTIA

Since the 1990s, four cholinesterase inhibitors and one N-methyl-D-aspartate (NMDA) antagonist were approved for use in the United States for slowing the progression of dementia. The first medication, tacrine (Cognex), is rarely prescribed because the newer cholinesterase inhibitors are safer and equally effective. Although no new medication has been developed since 2003, newer dosing options are available for several of these existing medications. A main difference between the two types of medications is that treatment with cholinesterase inhibitors usually begins early in the course of dementia and the NMDA antagonist is used alone or in combination with a cholinesterase inhibitor during moderate and later stages. Table 4.1 summarizes actions, doses, and common side effects of medications for dementia.

*Cholinesterase Inhibitors:* donepezil (Aricept), rivastigmine (Exelon), and galantamine (Razadyne, formerly called Reminyl). These medications:

- Increase levels of acetylcholine, a neurotransmitter that affects memory and cognition
- Are standard treatment to delay progression of symptoms of mild-to-moderate dementia; donepezil was recently approved for all stages of dementia
- Are similar in therapeutic effectiveness (i.e., modest improvement or delay in progression of symptoms)
- Have similar side effects: nausea, diarrhea, vomiting, anorexia, weight loss
- Have less common side effects such as vivid dreams or nightmares, which can be addressed by reducing the dose or avoiding bedtime administration
- May differ in individual response to therapeutic and adverse effects
- Are started at low dose and increased incrementally to prevent adverse effects and to reach optimal therapeutic levels

- Have been studied extensively for Alzheimer's disease, but are often used for other types of dementia because data about these conditions are limited
- Are less effective when anticholinergic medications are taken

Although many questions have been raised about the long-term therapeutic effectiveness of cholinesterase inhibitors, a recent review of studies found that benefits may last from 3 to 5 years and may be greater when treatment is started earlier (Wollen, 2010).

*N-methyl-D-aspartate antagonist*: memantine (Namenda). This medication:

- Regulates the level of the neurotransmitter glutamate in the brain, which is altered in dementia
- Is standard treatment of moderate-to-severe dementia, alone or in combination with a cholinesterase inhibitor
- Has the therapeutic effect of a modest improvement or delay in progression of symptoms for about 6 months
- Should be used cautiously in people with severe renal disease, or in combination with amantadine (Symmetrel) or dextromethorphan (Delsym)

=====*FAST FACTS in a NUTSHELL*

People with dementia typically begin taking a cholinesterase inhibitor during early or moderate stages and memantine is added to the regimen during a later stage.

**CLINICAL SNAPSHOT:** Mrs. H began taking donepezil when she was first diagnosed with dementia, but she experienced gastrointestinal effects and lost weight. The medication was discontinued and after 2 weeks she began using the rivastigmine patch, which she tolerated well. Two years later, memantine was added to her regimen.

## TABLE 4.1  Medications Approved for Dementia

| Medication | Action | Dose | Common Side Effects |
|---|---|---|---|
| donepezil (Aricept) | Prevents breakdown of acetylcholine in the brain | Begin with 5 mg once daily at bedtime; after 4–6 weeks, increase to 10 mg at bedtime as tolerated; after 3 months or more, increase to 23 mg for moderate to severe dementia | Nausea, vomiting, diarrhea |
| rivastigmine (Exelon) | Prevents breakdown of acetylcholine and butyrylcholine in the brain | *Oral* (with full meal): Begin with 1.5 mg twice daily; at 2–4 week intervals, increase to 3 mg, 4.5 mg, and 6 mg twice daily as tolerated *Transdermal* (rotate sites): Begin with 4.6 mg daily; after 4–6 weeks, increase to 9.5 mg | Nausea, vomiting, anorexia, diarrhea, weight loss, muscle weakness |
| galantamine (Razadyne) | Prevents breakdown of acetylcholine and stimulates nicotinic receptors to release acetylcholine in the brain | Begin with 4 mg twice daily with food; at 4–6 week intervals, increase to 8 mg and 12 mg twice daily as tolerated; extended release form can be taken once daily | Nausea, vomiting, anorexia, weight loss |
| memantine (Namenda) | Regulates glutamate activation and blocks toxic effects of excess glutamate | Begin with 5 mg once daily; at 1–2 weeks intervals, increase to 5 mg and 10 mg daily, then 10 mg twice daily as tolerated | Dizziness, headache, constipation, confusion |

## NURSING CONSIDERATIONS ABOUT MEDICATIONS FOR DEMENTIA

Nurses have many opportunities to teach about medications for dementia, particularly for people with mild dementia and for care partners of people with all stages of dementia. Some points to emphasize are:

- Many studies indicate that cholinesterase inhibitors have modest effects in delaying the progression of dementia.
- Medications are most effective when started early in the course of the condition.
- People with manifestations of dementia should be evaluated for appropriate medication management by a geriatrician or at a geriatric assessment program.
- As dementia progresses, medications should be re-evaluated.
- Donepezil is the only medication approved for all stages of dementia.
- Memantine is the only medication approved as an "add-on" to cholinesterase inhibitors for moderate to severe stages.
- Medications for dementia are started at low doses and increased gradually because adverse effects tend to diminish and the dose can be increased to therapeutic levels.
- It is important to follow the recommended titration doses and allow adequate time between dose adjustments.
- If compliance is difficult to achieve with pills, consider using transdermal patches (rivastigmine), once-daily dosing (donepezil, galantamine-ER), disintegrating sublingual tablets (donepezil), or a flavored liquid form (rivastigmine, memantine)
- If medications are not taken for several days, re-titration may be necessary.
- Because these medications slow the progression of symptoms but do not otherwise alter the course of dementia, it is difficult to evaluate their effectiveness.

=====*FAST FACTS in a NUTSHELL*

Address questions about medications for dementia during the usual course of providing care.

🌀 **CLINICAL SNAPSHOT:** Mrs. W is being admitted for rehabilitation following knee replacement surgery and she states, "I've been having memory problems for about a year and my doctor told me I should take a medication for Alzheimer's, but I haven't started because my friend took something for that and then she lost a lot of weight." You respond: "There are several medications that are helpful for Alzheimer's and they don't all have the same side effects. In fact, one of the medications can be used as a patch so it wouldn't affect your appetite or stomach. I suggest that you talk again with your doctor about trying one of these medications because they can slow the progression of your memory problem."

## CONSIDERATIONS FOR NON-ALZHEIMER'S DEMENTIA

As discussed in Chapter 1, more information is available for Alzheimer's disease than for other types of dementia, but information related to specific types of dementia is increasing rapidly. Considerations specific to management of non-Alzheimer's dementia that are pertinent to nursing care of people with dementia are summarized in Table 4.2.

## NONPRESCRIPTION AGENTS

As interest in complementary and alternative medicine (CAM) has grown during the past two decades, there has been increasing emphasis on improving cognitive function through nonprescription agents, such as herbs and vitamins.

**TABLE 4.2 Nursing Considerations Related to Medications for Non-Alzheimer's Dementia**

| Considerations for Non-Alzheimer's Dementia | Nursing Implications |
|---|---|
| Lewy body dementia increases sensitivity to adverse and therapeutic effects of many medications. Example: Risperidone and olanzapine are associated with higher incidence or exacerbation of extrapyramidal effects. | Use antipsychotics and benzodiazepines with caution; use very low doses; observe for adverse effects; if antipsychotics are necessary, quetiapine is the preferred drug; teach about avoiding prescription and nonprescription products with strong anticholinergic properties, including decongestants and antihistamines; assess for and document drug allergies and precautions. |
| People with Lewy body dementia may decompensate more when they have medical conditions. | Assess for physiologic disorders as soon as behavior changes are observed. |
| Even during mild stages, Lewy body dementia causes autonomic nervous system dysfunctions affecting swallowing, digestion, blood pressure, temperature regulation, and bowel and bladder control. | Carefully assess all aspects of functioning; teach about importance of appropriate and consistent medical management by a neurologist or other specialist. |
| Movement and balance disorders often occur early in Lewy body dementia. | Arrange for physical and occupational therapy to promote safe and optimal functioning. |
| Risk factors associated with vascular dementia should be addressed early and consistently, especially during mild and moderate stages. | Teach patients and care partners to talk with primary care practitioners about management of cardiovascular risk factors, including lipids, blood pressure, and low-dose aspirin. |

Health care professionals often are asked about these products, which are extensively marketed as beneficial not only for people with dementia, but also for all older adults. Table 4.3 is a guide to teaching about products that are widely advertised as "cognitive enhancers" or treatments for dementia.

## TABLE 4.3 Nonprescription Products Promoted for Dementia

| Product | Evidence | Precautions |
| --- | --- | --- |
| Ginkgo biloba | Studies of 120–160 mg daily have found improved cognition to a small degree in some people with dementia but no preventive effects. | May increase the risk for bleeding if taken with anticoagulants or nonsteroidal anti-inflammatory agents. |
| Vitamin E | Studies suggest that higher levels of Vitamin E *from food sources* (e.g., wheat germ oil, sunflower seeds, almonds, and sunflower or safflower oil) are associated with improved cognition. | More than 400 IU daily as a dietary supplement have been associated with serious adverse effects, including increased mortality. |
| Huperzine A | This plant extract increases acetylcholine in the brain and may be effective in delaying the progression of dementia, but more studies are needed. | Adverse effects include nausea, vomiting, diarrhea, sweating, restlessness, and blurred vision; contraindicated in people with seizure disorder. |
| Curcumin (turmeric) | This herb has many neuroprotective properties but studies related to dementia are inconclusive. | No known adverse effects. |
| Resveratrol | This natural substance found in red wine, peanuts, and other plants has beneficial health effects, but studies related to dementia are inconclusive. | Contraindicated in people with history of estrogen-sensitive tumors; may interact with blood thinners. |
| Panax ginseng | This herb has neuroprotective effects but studies related to dementia are inconclusive. | Insomnia and gastrointestinal effects may occur; may have hormone-like effects when used for more than 3 months. |
| Acetyl L-carnitine (ALCAR) | Some, but not all, studies found that this amino acid improved cognition and delayed progression of dementia. | Can interact with medications for hypothyroidism and seizure disorders. |

When teaching about nonprescription agents, incorporate the following points:

- Be sure to talk with your primary care practitioner about any nonprescription products you are using or considering using for health-related purposes.
- Obtain information about safety and efficacy of a product through reliable sources such as the National Center on Complementary and Alternative Medicine (nccam.nih.gov) or the Food and Drug Administration (www.fda.gov).
- Because dietary supplements are not regulated, products vary in quality and do not necessarily contain the advertised quantity of ingredients.
- Dietary supplements do not have standardized quantities of ingredients, so an accurate dose is difficult to determine.
- Herbs and all other biologically active products can have adverse effects as well as drug interactions.

═══════════════════════════════*FAST FACTS in a NUTSHELL*

Nurses have many opportunities to teach about nonprescription products for dementia.

**CLINICAL SNAPSHOT:** Mr. N, who is in the hospital for hip surgery, was recently diagnosed with dementia. When you are administering his donepezil he says "I've been taking this medicine for 6 months and I don't seem to be any better. My wife says that I should start taking Ginkgo, do you know anything about that?" You respond: "Although some studies indicate that Ginkgo may be helpful, it's important to talk with your primary care practitioner about this and to be aware of drug interactions if you do take it. Also, it's important to obtain it from a reliable source because the quality of those products varies."

## MEDICATIONS FOR MANAGEMENT OF DEMENTIA-RELATED SYMPTOMS

Medications are used for their direct effects on dementia and are used less commonly for the management of dementia-associated behaviors (as discussed extensively in Chapter 13). Despite concerns about using behavior-modifying medications for people with dementia, antipsychotics and antianxiety agents are sometimes necessary, especially in acute care settings. If these medications are deemed necessary, nurses can follow these guidelines:

- Use the lowest effective dose.
- Establish clear nursing criteria for using prn (as needed) medications (i.e., use only for patient safety or comfort, rather than for behaviors that are simply annoying).
- Frequently assess and document effects of medication.
- Assess for adverse effects, especially those that affect safety (e.g., increased fall risk, increased confusion).
- Assess optimal interval for administering prn medications.
- Frequently reassess the need for medications.
- If antianxiety or antipsychotic medications have been initiated in an acute care setting, provide information in discharge documents, including instructions for follow-up as appropriate (including considerations for not continuing after discharge).

## NONPHARMACOLOGIC INTERVENTIONS

Nurses caring for people with dementia as a secondary diagnosis can incorporate the following interventions to address cognitive deficits in their usual course of providing care:

- State your name when you initiate communication
- Make frequent casual references to the time of day, season of year, and so forth

- Make sure information on dry-erase boards in patient rooms is accurate and up to date
- Use simple written reminders about procedures and other scheduled activities
- Provide frequent reminders about using the call system for assistance
- Ask about pleasant memories and enjoyable activities (e.g., "Do you have a favorite memory about where you grew up?")
- Encourage use of simple relaxation practices (e.g., deep breathing, music)

In addition, nurses can incorporate interventions for safety, comfort, and physical needs (see Chapter 2) and interventions for addressing aspects of dementia discussed in Parts II, III, and IV of this book. Nurses can keep up to date on developments related to management of dementia by finding information from sites listed in the Resources in a Nutshell section.

## *RESOURCES in a NUTSHELL*

*Alzheimer's Association*
*alz.org*

*National Center for Complementary and Alternative Medicine (NCCAM)*
*nccam.nih.gov*

# Caring for the Person
# With Dementia

# 5

## Providing Person-Centered Care for People With Dementia

### INTRODUCTION

*A major shift has been occurring from the traditional medical model of care for people with dementia to a model of person-centered care that focuses on interventions to promote comfort and to maintain the best quality of life for people with dementia and their families and care partners. Person-centered care is consistent with holistic nursing care because nurses routinely assess a patient— including all aspects of body, mind, and spirit—and address individualized needs. Nurses can use these same skills to identify and address individualized needs of people with dementia and their care partners. The main difference is that people with dementia may not be able to clearly communicate their needs. Thus, a detective-like approach may be needed to identify and address their needs. In a nutshell, find the person behind the dementia and relate to this person in a caring way. This chapter discusses principles of person-centered care and identifies ways in which nurses can apply these strategies when caring for people with dementia.*

In this chapter, you will learn:

1. A description of person-centered care
2. How to apply person-centered care during your usual care for people with dementia
3. Resources for culturally appropriate care

## COMPONENTS OF PERSON-CENTERED CARE

Since the 1990s, dementia-care experts have been advocating that interventions, including all interactions, focus on the "personhood" of the person with dementia. This emphasis is necessary because dementia is characterized by progressive losses and people with dementia gradually lose their relationships with self, others, and their environment. As people with dementia lose their sense of self and increasingly depend on others for all their needs, care partners need to affirm and strengthen the individual's sense of self as much as possible. This is accomplished through a person-centered approach to care.

Tom Kitwood, a gerontology professor in England, promulgated a model of person-centered care that has become widely accepted as a standard of care. Key concepts of this model include:

- The person being cared for is the center of all actions and decisions.
- Care is focused on the whole person, not just on the diagnosis, symptoms, or physical functioning.
- Interventions are directed toward maintaining and promoting comfort, dignity, respect, and a sense of wellness.
- Care plans emphasize strengths and abilities rather than deficits.
- Level of assistance is based on an assessment of the person's needs and abilities (i.e., not too much, not too little).

- Care plans identify and address emotional needs and personal preferences.
- Care settings are designed to promote positive social environments.
- The institutional environment needs to be adapted to compensate for the needs of people with dementia.

Nurses can suggest that families find information about long-term care facilities that incorporate person-centered care through the Internet sites listed in the Resources in a Nutshell at the end of this chapter.

Although Kitwood's model was developed specifically for long-term care of people with dementia, the principles can be applied in any care setting. Examples of ways in which these principles can be incorporated during usual nursing care include the following:

- Ask the person with dementia or their care partners about likes/dislikes related to food, personal care, and preferred name.
- Notice the greeting cards, flowers, and other signs of love and friendship that are in the patient's room and ask about the sender.
- Ask open-ended questions about social and work interests: What activities do you do to keep your life interesting? What kind of work did you do? Where did you live as a child?
- Find out if the person needs demonstrations or "getting started actions" to initiate an activity. Example: The person may need a guiding hand before he or she can get out of a chair.
- Let the person know what you are going to do before you start the activity, but do not be condescending. Example: Do not say "We are going to take our pills."

=====FAST FACTS in a NUTSHELL

It is helpful to incorporate information about likes and dislikes into care plans to facilitate care of people with dementia.

**CLINICAL SNAPSHOT:** When Mrs. H, who has moderate dementia, is admitted for pneumonia, her daughter says she has difficulty chewing meat and hates the usual mechanical soft diet. You ask about food preferences and document that she enjoys casserole-type foods and will always eat sandwiches made with smooth peanut butter and jelly.

## UNDERSTANDING THE EXPERIENCE OF PEOPLE WITH DEMENTIA

A key component of providing person-centered care is to develop an understanding of how people with dementia experience and respond to their condition. One way of seeing the world through the perspective of people with dementia is to imagine that you have just arrived in a foreign country where you do not understand the language or recognize any of the people. This image illustrates that people with dementia may not be able to understand complex verbal or written instructions, but they will notice nonverbal communication and interpret this in their unique ways. Another way of developing empathy for people with dementia is to talk with people who have mild and moderate dementia about their feelings and experiences, as discussed in Chapter 6.

Although nurses caring for people with dementia as a secondary diagnosis focus their care on the primary diagnoses, they can identify and address the needs and feelings related to dementia during the course of their regular care. For example, nurses can learn about the experiences of people with dementia by asking simple questions such as "So what techniques do you use to cope with your memory problems?" Some answers to this kind of question, as verbalized by people with mild and moderate dementia, have been documented by the Alzheimer's Society (2008, 2010) in Great Britain, as follows:

- I allow myself to focus on the pain and fear but then I move away from the sad focus.
- I try to do something that I can still do—not as well as before—but something that I can still do.
- It's very important to laugh and enjoy a joke or pleasantries with people.
- I slow down and reset my expectations because expecting that you can be who you used to be is just a recipe for pain and sadness.
- I curse it every now and then and that helps.
- Inertia is a serious problem with me and sometimes I seem glued to my chair.
- I think it would be better if I did not drive and it is much better that I make that decision for myself.
- When I have to start asking for help, I want to be consulted and have some say in my independence.
- When I am unable to verbalize what I want, it's helpful that my wife displays multiple options and allows me to choose one.
- I think it would be nice if people gave you the courtesy of time to finish what you are trying to say.
- It's somewhat humiliating to have to ask for help and adjust your schedule to someone else's when you're used to running your own life.

By asking this kind of question during the course of usual care, nurses communicate that dementia is a chronic condition that requires coping skills. This kind of question also communicates that you are interested in learning about the person's response to dementia. Moreover, it provides an opportunity to elicit information about the person's experience, so you can identify and address their needs and feelings.

======= *FAST FACTS in a NUTSHELL*

There are many opportunities to identify and address the needs and feelings of people with dementia during the usual course of providing care.

**CLINICAL SNAPSHOT:** During the admission assessment, Mrs. C tells you that she uses the rivastigmine (Exelon) patch because she was recently diagnosed with dementia. In response to your question about how she copes, she says "Sometimes I feel pretty lonely and stupid because my bridge group doesn't want me there anymore and I used to have lunch and cards with them every week." You respond: "I'm sure it's hard to deal with dementia and I appreciate you talking about your experiences. Did you know that the Alzheimer's Association has social, support, and educational programs for people with dementia? I can give you their phone number so you can call them after you get home."

## PROVIDING CULTURALLY APPROPRIATE CARE

Because person-centered care inherently is culturally appropriate, identify and address cultural aspects that influence people with dementia and their care partners. Cultural background includes race and ethnicity, as well as characteristics associated with religion, education, socioeconomic status, sexual orientation, and other influential factors. Cultural factors—on the part of the nurse, the person with dementia, and all care partners—are likely to influence all the following aspects of care for people with dementia:

- Assessment of mental status
- Perceptions of cognitive changes
- Interpretation of dementia-related behaviors
- Beliefs about causes of mental changes
- Expectations related to caregiver roles within the family
- Acceptance of caregiver resources from outside the family
- Verbal communication (e.g., primary and secondary languages spoken and comprehended, which can change or fluctuate during the course of dementia)
- Nonverbal communication (e.g., touch, personal space, eye contact, facial expressions)
- Discussions about treatment options, including care during advanced dementia
- Management of pain and other symptoms
- Attitudes toward health care decisions (e.g., informed consent, health care proxies, advance directives)
- Acceptance of referrals for hospice, palliative care, and support services for the person with dementia and his or her care partners
- Acceptance of different health care practices, including use and acceptance of pharmacologic and nonpharmacologic interventions
- Use of various health care practitioners (e.g., physicians, nurse practitioners, herbalists, and complementary and alternative practitioners)

Although it is unrealistic to expect to be knowledgeable about specific characteristics of all cultural groups, it is possible to be aware of the ways in which these characteristics influence care of people with dementia. Nurses can also incorporate culturally appropriate interventions, particularly with regard to referrals for services, into care of the individual and his or her discharge plans. For example, obtain health education materials in other languages from culturally specific organizations listed in the Resources in a Nutshell at the end of this chapter.

## FAST FACTS in a NUTSHELL

There are many opportunities to incorporate cultur-ally appropriate interventions as an integral part of person-centered care for people with dementia and their families.

**CLINICAL SNAPSHOT:** Mrs. S's daughter confides that she is overwhelmed with caring for her mother, who lives with her and has advanced dementia. Her mother was born in Puerto Rico and used to speak English but now she understands only Spanish. You arrange for the hospital social worker to talk with her about local re-sources of the Alzheimer's Association, which provide culturally specific services for Hispanics.

## RESOURCES in a NUTSHELL

### Long-Term Care Facilities That Incorporate Person-Centered Care

*Advancing Excellence in America's Nursing Homes*
*www.nhqualitycampaign.org*

*Center for Excellence in Assisted Living*
*www.theceal.org*

*Pioneer Network*
*www.pioneernetwork.net*

### Dementia Information in Other Languages

*Alzheimer's Association*
*www.alz.org/diversity/overview.asp*

*(continued)*

*(continued)*

**Alzheimer's Disease International**
*www.alz.co.uk/other-languages*

**MedlinePlus**
*www.nlm.nih.gov/medlineplus/languages/dementia.html*

# 6

## Caring for the Person With Mild Dementia

### INTRODUCTION

*As noted in Chapter 1, the diagnosis of dementia is based on a comprehensive evaluation of cognitive changes that have developed over months or years, except in the relatively few cases when the dementia is the consequence of a stroke or other major medical event. Thus, the onset of mild dementia occurs gradually and only the person with dementia and his or her close contacts notice the early manifestations. People with mild dementia can maintain a relatively safe and independent level of functioning, but they need to compensate for cognitive deficits. They may be able to live alone with help from support resources or they may be living with their spouse or family or in an assisted living facility.*

*Nurses can recognize mild dementia under any of the following circumstances:*

- *The person or care partner reports cognitive impairments that have been occurring during previous months or years and interfere with daily functioning.*

> - *Nurses observe significant cognitive impairments that are not associated with another diagnosis (e.g., delirium, depression).*
> - *A diagnosis of dementia has been documented and the person is functioning at a relatively independent level.*
>
> *In either of the first two circumstances, nursing responsibilities focus on assessment issues, and in all circumstances, nurses caring for people with mild dementia focus on safety issues. In addition, nurses provide person-centered care by addressing the emotional needs of people with mild dementia.*

In this chapter, you will learn:

1. Assessment issues and related nursing strategies
2. Common safety concerns and related nursing strategies
3. How to address emotional needs

## ASSESSMENT ISSUES

Some people with dementia are acutely aware of the earliest changes, whereas others have little or no insight or awareness at any time during the course of this condition. Thus, as a nurse who cares for people with mild dementia, it will become apparent that some patients will offer information about having dementia and others will adamantly insist that they have no cognitive impairments despite evidence to the contrary. A common assessment issue is that people with mild dementia may object to obtaining an evaluation, but this does not mean that such a discussion should be avoided. Rather, address the issue in a similar manner to suggesting an assessment of other aspects of functioning.

This can be accomplished by asking patients or their families and care partners about the onset and duration of these changes and about any evaluation of these changes.

=======================*FAST FACTS in a NUTSHELL*

During the course of usual nursing care, discuss observations about the person's memory (or other aspects of cognition) and ask if this has been addressed in any medical evaluation.

🌀 **CLINICAL SNAPSHOT:** When you perform the initial nursing assessment on Mrs. T, who is being admitted for upper GI bleeding, you note that she repeatedly asks the same questions and seems to give inaccurate information in response to your questions. You say, "I noticed that you have some trouble with your memory, have you talked with your doctor about this so it can be evaluated?"

In some situations, dementia may have been diagnosed but not documented as a current problem—particularly when the focus of care is on other conditions (e.g., in hospital settings). In a community-based setting where there is little documentation of medical conditions, ask the person to sign a release of information to obtain pertinent medical information. If the person is not aware of a diagnosis of dementia—or does not remember that dementia has been diagnosed—it is important to obtain permission to talk with care partners and involved health care professionals about any evaluations. Ask if the person has any written reports from assessment programs that he or she is willing to share. If the person is taking one of the dementia-specific medications discussed in Chapter 4, ask about the related diagnosis. Use Table 6.1 as a guide to addressing assessment issues commonly associated with mild dementia.

## TABLE 6.1 Assessment Issues and Related Nursing Strategies

| Assessment Issues | Nursing Strategies |
| --- | --- |
| Different levels of awareness of cognitive impairments | Ask open-ended questions about changes in ability to remember things or manage usual responsibilities; assess whether the reported level of functioning is consistent with objective assessment findings. |
| Attributing significant changes to "normal aging" | Emphasize that there are many conditions that affect cognitive functioning for people at all ages and that it is important to identify those that can be treated. |
| Inability to obtain accurate information about cognitive changes from the person experiencing the changes | Obtain permission to talk with a close companion or family member and explain that this is necessary for an accurate and complete assessment; create opportunities for family members to express concerns about changes in the person's functioning. |
| Family members express concern about cognitive changes but the person with mild dementia has no awareness of impairments or denies the need for assessment | Identify an aspect of functioning that the person acknowledges is problematic or talk with the person about the concerns noted by the family and encourage the person to have this evaluated at a geriatric assessment program so treatable conditions can be identified. |
| Not enough time to address assessment issues | Document concerns and teach about the importance of having cognitive changes evaluated as part of the discharge plan. |

## ═════════════════════════════*FAST FACTS in a NUTSHELL*

Many strategies can be used to facilitate an evaluation of people with manifestations of mild dementia (Table 6.1).

## COMMON SAFETY CONCERNS

People with mild dementia typically live alone or with a spouse, partner, or family member and they require supervision or minimal assistance when performing complex activities. Safety concerns that commonly occur during mild dementia include driving, meal preparation, and accurate management of finances and medications. When dementia is mild, these concerns usually do not pose major threats; however, they are likely to present additional risks to safety as the dementia progresses, so be proactive in addressing these issues.

Although inpatient settings may present limited opportunities to address safety issues related to home settings, home safety risks can be addressed in discharge plans. Nurses in acute care settings, including emergency rooms, need to assess whether cognitive impairments have contributed to the presenting problem. For example, mild dementia can compromise the ability to take medications accurately, and this may have led to the emergency medical condition (as described in the Clinical Snapshot at the end of this chapter). Nurses in community-based settings have opportunities to identify risks for safe functioning and to teach about strategies to reduce the risk.

Safety concerns can be assessed by asking the person about any difficulties in performing daily activities and by obtaining information from family members and care partners. When safety concerns are noted, you can teach about simple strategies to diminish the risk, as detailed in Table 6.2.

===============*FAST FACTS in a NUTSHELL*

Use assessment questions to identify "red flags" for potential safety concerns.

🔹 **CLINICAL SNAPSHOT:** Mr. B's daughter tells you she is wondering if her father is safe living alone because he has dementia and he drives to church and the grocery store. You ask about all of the following: recent car accidents, dents in the car, burned pots and pans, ability to take medications as prescribed, ability to initiate phone calls if he needs help, and evidence of bills not being paid or money that cannot be accounted for.

### TABLE 6.2 Safety Concerns and Related Nursing Strategies

| Safety Concern | Nursing Strategies to Diminish the Risk |
| --- | --- |
| Unsafe driving | Suggest that a formal driving evaluation be performed by a specially trained occupational therapist; emphasize that the person may qualify for a driving rehabilitation program or may be safe with restrictions on driving; refer to appropriate resources listed at end of this chapter. |
| Difficulty managing medications | Teach about the many medication management systems that can be used, ranging from readily available daily dosing containers to more complex automated 28-day systems; refer to appropriate resources listed at end of this chapter. |
| Unsafe use of stove | Consider installing shutoff valves or removing knobs; use electric tea kettle with automatic shutoff for boiling water; encourage use of microwave oven if this can be done safely. |
| Unawareness of spoiled food | Arrange for weekly checking of food. |
| Risk for financial exploitation; inability to manage bill paying | Teach about the importance of establishing a financial power of attorney and having a trustworthy person assist as necessary with financial management. |

==========*FAST FACTS in a NUTSHELL*

In any clinical setting, nurses have opportunities to assess for or ask about safety concerns and suggest interventions (Table 6.2).

## EMOTIONAL NEEDS

Even for the most well-adjusted person, the diagnosis of dementia is a life-altering event with major implications, not only for the person with dementia but also for those who are close to that person. In recent years, people with mild dementia have shared their experiences through books, films, blogs, interviews, and other publicly available media, and health care professionals and Alzheimer's advocacy groups have published references and reports on the expressed needs of people with mild dementia. An overriding theme expressed by people with mild dementia is that myths and misconceptions lead to stigma and misunderstanding, which affect their relationships with family, friends, colleagues, and health care professionals. Expressed needs of people with mild dementia that are pertinent to nurses providing person-centered care include:

- Talking about their condition but not being stereotyped
- Having people listen to them as individuals
- Expressing feelings about the effects of their condition
- Having people recognize and respect both their abilities and limitations
- Being asked about how they cope with the challenges of their condition
- Receiving support from professionals about their positive coping mechanisms
- Maintaining independent functioning in daily activities
- Talking about the ways in which others can be helpful
- Participating in support and educational groups

- Maintaining continuity with past interests, relationships, and social roles
- Developing new interests that are consistent with current abilities
- Connecting with others who experience early-stage dementia
- Teaching others about their disease
- Finding reliable information and resources

Additional information about these expressed needs is provided in the Resources in a Nutshell section at the end of this chapter.

═══════════════════════════════*FAST FACTS in a NUTSHELL*

People with mild dementia consistently express the need to be recognized as individuals and receive support from health care professionals to strengthen their coping abilities.

**CLINICAL SNAPSHOT:** Mrs. T tells you she has been diagnosed with Alzheimer's disease and now her friends do not want her in their bridge club. You respond: "I'm sure you have lots to offer in other ways because you are so friendly and have traveled a lot. Would you be willing to participate in the 'Memory Lane' group that meets here every Wednesday afternoon after lunch?"

A practical way of addressing emotional needs of people with mild dementia is to ask simple and emphatic questions during the course of your usual nursing care. *Living Your Best with Early-Stage Alzheimer's* by Lisa Snyder (Sunrise River Press, North Branch, MN) is an excellent resource for in-depth exploration of issues and coping strategies that can be used by people with mild dementia and health care professionals.

Some of the discussion questions from this book, which are listed in Exhibit 6.1, can be used when asking people with mild dementia about their experiences and feelings.

In recent years, Alzheimer's Associations, which are available in every community, have increasingly addressed the

---

**Exhibit 6.1**    Questions for Discussion
for People With Mild Dementia

How did you react to the diagnosis of Alzheimer's?

How have your loved ones or friends reacted to your diagnosis and what kinds of reactions are helpful or unhelpful?

What are your strengths and abilities?

What memory-loss and coping strategies do you use?

Have you or your care partner observed any ways that Alzheimer's has affected your safety? If so, what modifications have you made?

What ideas do you have for maximizing your independence and safety?

Do you have a spiritual faith or practice that helps you cope? Have your beliefs been affected by the onset of Alzheimer's?

Are you able to communicate effectively with your health care team? If not, what are the challenges?

How do you feel about having a loved one with you during your appointments?

Have you been able to get answers to questions you have about Alzheimer's?

*Source:* Adapted from Snyder (2010). Used with permission.

needs of people with mild dementia. As part of ongoing care or discharge plans, nurses can suggest that people with mild dementia consider participating in support and educational groups, either in person or through Internet resources. At a minimum, provide the phone number of the local Alzheimer's Association and encourage the person to explore this resource. Explain that even if the person has not been diagnosed with Alzheimer's, this organization is an excellent source of information and provides support resources about cognitive impairments and all types of dementia. In addition, provide a copy of the Resources in a Nutshell section at the end of this chapter and encourage people with dementia and their care partners to explore these resources.

## ════════════════════════════*FAST FACTS in a NUTSHELL*

Nurses caring for people with mild dementia in any setting can ask them about their feelings and experiences, with emphasis on their ways of coping (Exhibit 6.1)

🌀 CLINICAL SNAPSHOT: NURSING CARE FOR A PERSON WITH MILD DEMENTIA IN THE EMERGENCY ROOM

Mrs. S, a 78-year-old widow who lives alone, was brought to the emergency room after she passed out while playing cards with friends. She is alert and responsive and oriented x3. Her medications include furosemide (Lasix) every morning, ramipril (Altace) twice daily, metoprolol (Lopressor) twice daily, and potassium powder effervescent (KLOR-CON/EF). All diagnostic tests are within normal, except for a serum

*(continued)*

(*continued*)

potassium of 2.8 mEq/L. When you ask about her medications, she reports that she takes one water pill and two heart pills in the morning, and sometimes an extra water pill in the afternoon if her feet seem swollen. Upon further questioning, she tells you that she thinks she's been taking the extra water pill recently but she really can't remember how often. You specifically ask about the potassium powder and she states "Oh, I usually forget to take that because it's not in the compartment with my other pills." When Mrs. S's daughter arrives, you ask if she has noticed changes in her mother's cognitive abilities and she reports that her mother has been forgetting appointments and has not been paying her bills as usual. The daughter has been concerned about these changes and has considered having an evaluation at the geriatric assessment program. You teach Mrs. S and her daughter about the importance of following through with the geriatric assessment appointment and you suggest that Mrs. S allow her daughter to oversee her medication system.

## RESOURCES in a NUTSHELL

### *Alzheimer's Association*
*www.alz.org*

- Information about educational and support services for people with mild dementia and their families and care partners
- Information about medical alert devices specifically for people with dementia

*Family Caregiver Alliance, National Center on Caregiving*

*caregiver.org*

• Fact Sheet: Alzheimer's Disease, Early Stage

*Perspectives,* free quarterly newsletter published by University of California, San Diego Shiley-Marcos Alzheimer's Disease Research Center; email requests to:

*lsnyder@ucsd.edu*

• Addresses concerns, reflections, and coping skills of individuals with Alzheimer's or a related disorder
• Provides up-to-date information, explores relevant topics, provides a discussion forum, and builds bridges among people with memory loss around the world

## Books

• *How to Live Well With Early Alzheimer's* by Deborah Mitchell, New York, NY: St. Martin's Press, 2010.
• *Living Your Best With Early-Stage Alzheimer's* by Lisa Snyder, North Branch, MN: Sunrise River Press, 2010.

## Audiovisuals

• *The Forgetting: A Portrait of Alzheimer's,* pbs/org/theforgetting/experience/index.html (view or download the transcript in English or Spanish)
• *I Have Alzheimer's Disease: Shared Experiences,* www.alzheimer.ca (listen to personal experiences of people with mild dementia in English or French)

# 7

# Caring for the Person With Moderate Dementia

## INTRODUCTION

*Moderate dementia is best described as the stage between early and advanced dementia. There are no clear boundaries among any of the stages because, although dementia progresses gradually, the course is not necessarily a consistent downhill path. Rather, people with dementia fluctuate in their functioning because of changes in health status, environment, care partners, and other conditions. This chapter focuses on nursing issues that are most closely associated with moderate dementia, but the information in most other chapters of the book is also pertinent to this stage of dementia.*

In this chapter, you will learn:

1. Characteristics of moderate dementia
2. How to facilitate decisions about care
3. How to promote safe and independent functioning

## CHARACTERISTICS OF MODERATE DEMENTIA

Reisberg's (1986) widely used scale for Functional Assessment of Alzheimer's Disease (FAST) describes characteristics of moderate and moderately severe dementia as:

- Obvious cognitive deficits (e.g., disorientation, significant short-term memory impairment)
- Difficulty remembering names of familiar people
- Unable to manage complex daily tasks without supervision or assistance
- Gradual loss of ability to perform activities of daily living (dressing, bathing, toileting)
- Development of urinary incontinence
- Development of bowel incontinence

These changes usually develop slowly over several years, or they may develop more rapidly if there are significant medical events, such as stroke or major surgery. In addition, a major change in support, such as loss of a significant care partner, can precipitate a rapid decline in functioning. In these situations, the person may seem to move rapidly from early to moderate dementia but the underlying disease process may actually be stable.

═══════════════════════════════*FAST FACTS in a NUTSHELL*

A person with early dementia may appear to move quickly to moderate dementia due to a major change in caregiver support.

**CLINICAL SNAPSHOT:** After Mrs. C's husband of 56 years died, her children noted that she was easily confused, did not remember what day it was, did not take her daily medications, forgot to eat, did not bathe, and was unsafe living alone. When they assessed the situation, they realized that their father had provided so much supervision and assistance that her early dementia was well hidden. They also found out that she had been taking galantamine (Razadyne) but had not told them about this.

## FACILITATING DECISIONS ABOUT CARE

People with dementia experience a wide range of emotions and behaviors that includes loss, fear, shame, anger, sadness, frustration, loneliness, depression, uncertainty, uselessness, self-blame, diminished affect, and withdrawal from challenging activities. These responses can be intense during the moderate stage as the person with dementia and his or her care partners experience the progression of changes. Because people with moderate dementia require more assistance with daily activities, they and their care partners face difficult decisions. Decisions about living arrangements usually arise for people who do not live with someone who can assume the necessary caregiving role. Decisions about support for caregivers arise in situations where family is expected to assume caregiving roles. These decisions are often associated with conflicts about independence versus safety and self-determination versus allowing others to make decisions. The process becomes very complex when the person with dementia does not have the insight and capacity to make safe and reasonable choices. During this phase, families, care partners, and people with dementia often seek advice from nurses. This is appropriate because nurses are skilled in holistically assessing and addressing needs, but it also is time consuming and challenging. Nurses can assist with these decisions by:

- Using Table 6.1 as a guide to assess safety concerns that arise during early dementia and continue through moderate dementia

- Using Table 7.1 as a guide to assess functioning
- Initiating referrals for assistance with complex decisions, as discussed in the next section

**TABLE 7.1  Assessment Issues and Related Nursing Actions**

| Assessment of Functioning | Nursing Actions |
| --- | --- |
| Cognitive abilities | Use cognitive assessment tools (e.g., mini-mental status examination); refer for geriatric assessment; assess memory, decision making, and other cognitive functions during all interactions; document all findings |
| Emotional aspects | Use screening tool for depression; ask about feelings and coping skills related to dementia; ask about spiritual/religious needs |
| Ability to call for help | Assess ability to use call light; assess or ask care partners about ability to initiate phone calls unassisted; assess ability to learn about emergency call system |
| Personal care activities | Assess grooming, bathing, oral care, and nail care; refer for occupational therapy if appropriate |
| Mobility | Assess balance, walking, and transferring; observe the person's interactions with the environment; refer for physical therapy if appropriate |
| Bowel and bladder control | Assess for ongoing or intermittent urinary or fecal incontinence; refer for evaluations as indicated (including checking for urinary tract infection); assess for constipation or fecal impaction; assess factors that increase the risk for incontinence (e.g., inaccessibility of toileting facility, relying on others for assistance) |
| Social supports | Ask about changes in social contacts (e.g., Are there enjoyable activities that you no longer do?); ask about transportation limitations |

In addition, nurses can teach families and care partners about interventions to promote safe and independent functioning, as discussed in the last section of this chapter.

## FAST FACTS in a NUTSHELL

Nurses can facilitate referrals for other services for assessments and recommendations.

**CLINICAL SNAPSHOT:** You are caring for Ms. R, who has been admitted for knee replacement surgery and has dementia as a secondary diagnosis. Upon admission, her hair was greasy and unkempt, she had a strong body odor and bad breath, and her clothes were soiled. She told you she lived alone and "I can take care of myself as I always have." You request an occupational therapy assessment and you arrange for the social worker to meet with Ms. R and her niece, who lives nearby and provides assistance with transportation and grocery shopping.

Nurses do not always have the skills or time to facilitate decisions about care of people with dementia, but they can refer for social worker assistance. Nurses also can suggest that families explore the wide range of caregiving resources and living arrangements, including assisted living, senior apartments with additional services, and specialized dementia care facilities. In addition, nurses can provide contact information (see the Resources in a Nutshell at the end of this chapter) for the following types of resources to assist with these decisions:

- Geriatric assessment programs for comprehensive multidisciplinary assessment and recommendations
- Geriatric care managers for initial and ongoing assistance with decisions about appropriate care

- Alzheimer's Association information hotline for advice about local resources
- Eldercare Locator for information about appropriate local resources

Nurses can emphasize that the increasing focus on person-centered care has prompted the development of holistic models of care for people with dementia. Care partners can find information about facilities that provide person-centered care at the web sites listed in the Resources in a Nutshell section at the end of Chapter 5.

═══════════════════════════════*FAST FACTS in a NUTSHELL*

Nurses can provide information about resources to assist with decisions about care issues, including conflicts related to safety versus independence.

🔄 CLINICAL SNAPSHOT: Mr. P's son confides that he thinks his father should move to an assisted living facility, but his father will not discuss this because he is "fiercely independent and stubborn as well." You provide contact information about local geriatric assessment programs and care managers and urge him to call. You emphasize that staff in these programs are happy to discuss the situation and can arrange for an assessment and recommendations.

## PROMOTING SAFE AND INDEPENDENT FUNCTIONING

An important challenge in caring for persons with moderate dementia is to implement strategies that promote safe and independent functioning (Table 7.2). Nurses have key roles in modifying environments as much as possible and in teaching about interventions that families and care partners can use.

## TABLE 7.2  Nursing Actions to Promote Safe and Independent Functioning

| Functional Aspect | Nursing Actions |
| --- | --- |
| Vision | Annual eye examinations; up-to-date prescription glasses; keep eyeglasses clean; optimal lighting; magnifying aids |
| Hearing | Hearing evaluation; use of hearing aid or amplifying device; assist as necessary with hearing aid care, insertion, and secure storage; good communication techniques |
| Memory and cognition | Accurate information on orientation boards; visibility of clocks and calendars; photos and other reminders of family and caring relationships |
| Personal care | Provide reminders and assist as necessary, but allow as much independence as possible; arrange for manicures, pedicures, and podiatry; arrange personal care items in a visible and uncluttered place in the order in which they are used; leave a toothbrush with toothpaste on it on the sink |
| Mobility | Assistive devices as recommended; physical therapy; group exercise programs (including tai chi); individual assistance for safety |
| Bowel and bladder control | Individualized toileting plan for maximum independence but minimal risk for incontinence; interventions to prevent constipation |
| General safety and functioning | Visual cues to designate important places (e.g., toilet, refrigerator); simple cues for operating thermostats, appliances, radios, televisions, and so forth |
| Usual environment | Keep the environment simple and uncluttered; keep medications, cleaning solutions, and any poisonous chemicals in inaccessible places |
| Wayfinding difficulties | Enroll in a protective program, such as the Safe Return program sponsored by the Alzheimer's Association; carry identification |

# FAST FACTS in a NUTSHELL

Nurses have many opportunities to teach about interventions to promote safe and independent functioning.

**CLINICAL SNAPSHOT:** You are caring for Mr. T after his cardiac surgery, and you observe that his eyeglasses look old and the side pieces are taped. He has a secondary diagnosis of dementia and lives in an assisted living facility. He cannot report information about his vision or eye examinations, but you assess that he cannot read the instructions about postsurgical care that were provided for him. When you meet with his daughter to discuss discharge plans, you find out that he has not had his eyes examined for at least 4 years. You emphasize that an annual eye examination is especially important for people with dementia because accurate sensory input is essential for compensating for cognitive deficits.

# RESOURCES in a NUTSHELL

*Alzheimer's Association*
www.alz.org

*Eldercare Locator*
www.eldercare.gov

*National Association of Professional Geriatric Care Managers*
www.caremanager.org

# 8

# Caring for the Person With Advanced Dementia

## INTRODUCTION

As discussed in Chapter 5, person-centered care focuses on comfort and quality of life for people with dementia and their care partners, and this focus becomes increasingly more important as dementia progresses to the advanced and terminal stage. During this phase, people with dementia have limited ability to express their needs and are no longer able to participate in decisions about care. Nurses in all settings have major roles in providing direct care to people with advanced dementia and in supporting and advising care partners regarding decisions about care. This chapter focuses on nursing issues that are most closely associated with advanced dementia, but the information in many other chapters is also pertinent to this stage of dementia.

In this chapter, you will learn:

1. Characteristics of advanced dementia
2. How to address decisions about care
3. How to address feeding and eating difficulties
4. Issues related to end-of-life care
5. Nursing care for comfort during advance dementia

# CHARACTERISTICS OF ADVANCED DEMENTIA

Dementia is a life-limiting condition and a leading cause of death; however, its course can last as long as 20 years, with an average of 40% of the time spent in the advanced stage (Arrighi, Neumann, Lieberburg, & Townsend, 2010). Advanced dementia has been described as "a steady prolonged dwindling," characterized by a gradual increase in frailty and advanced disability (van der Steen, 2010). As with other stages of dementia, there is no line of demarcation indicating that the person has advanced dementia. At some point during this stage, people who do not die of other causes become terminally ill because of dementia. Characteristics of advanced dementia are described in Table 8.1.

**TABLE 8.1  Characteristics of Advanced Dementia**

| Feature | Examples |
| --- | --- |
| Cognition | Unaware of surroundings<br>Unable to recognize familiar people<br>Severely impaired memory<br>Severely impaired judgment and decision making |
| Communication | Extremely limited verbal communication<br>Few intelligible words<br>Unable to comprehend and follow instructions<br>Eventually unable to smile<br>Unable to verbally express needs or symptoms of pain or distress |
| Functional level | Unable to perform activities of daily living, including eating, hygiene, toileting, and dressing<br>Unsteady and deteriorating gait, eventually bedridden<br>Unable to perform purposeful actions<br>Eventually becomes totally incontinent of bladder and bowel |
| Sleep and activity level | Shows little or no interest in activities<br>Disrupted and inconsistent sleep patterns<br>Eventually may sleep all or most of the time |

*(continued)*

**TABLE 8.1** *(continued)*

| Feature | Examples |
|---|---|
| Nutrition | Loss of appetite, forgetting to eat<br>Difficulty with chewing and swallowing<br>Risk of aspiration<br>Weight loss |
| Emotions | Loss of ability to verbally communicate<br>Presumed awareness of emotions communicated by others<br>May have heightened awareness of nonverbal communication from others<br>Presumed nonverbal expressions of emotions and needs |
| Medical complications | Increased incidence of seizures, pneumonia, dehydration, infection, electrolyte imbalances, and metabolic disturbances |
| Safety concerns | Unintentional self-harm caused by falls or poor fluid and nutritional intake |
| Behavioral issues | Hallucinations, loss of contact with reality<br>Nonaggressive agitation<br>Distressing and repetitive vocalization (yelling, moaning, crying)<br>Diminished ability to pace or wander, but increased risk of falls if ambulatory or able to get out of chair or bed |

*FAST FACTS in a NUTSHELL*

Advanced dementia lasts for several years and is characterized by a gradual loss of all physical functioning and the ability to express needs.

## DECISIONS ABOUT GOALS OF TREATMENT

During all phases of dementia, goals of care focus on quality of life, but during the early and moderate phases, goals also focus on curative and disease-modifying interventions for dementia as well as concomitant conditions. Because advanced dementia, like other phases, progresses gradually and lasts for several years, decisions about treatment goals are ongoing. People with advanced dementia are no longer able to participate in decisions about goals for their care, so families, health care proxies, and other care partners assume responsibility. Ideally, all legal issues need to be addressed when the person with dementia is able to participate in decisions, so that surrogate decision makers have guidelines to follow. Chapter 15 provides information about legal and ethical issues related to health care decisions for people with dementia. Even when advance directives are in place, surrogate decision makers and all care partners—including nurses—experience many emotional conflicts and ethical dilemmas because of the shift in goals. Factors that contribute to this challenge include:

- Simple daily activities become associated with health risks (e.g., difficulty chewing and swallowing increases the risk for aspiration pneumonia, and impaired balance and mobility increase the risk for falls), so decisions focus on freedom and pleasure versus potential harm.
- Even when guidelines are clear, surrogate decision makers often express discomfort because they feel they are "playing God."
- It is difficult to determine the onset of advanced dementia as an end-of-life condition.

In these situations, nurses can emphasize that the surrogate decision maker is acting out of love and concern by advocating for what the person with dementia wants. Additional roles of nurses include:

- Providing nursing input in interdisciplinary teams to discuss clinical issues
- Providing information about evidence-based guidelines for decisions

- Reviewing advance directives as the person's condition changes
- Assisting with discussions about advance directives
- Communicating with families and care partners about advance directives
- Documenting up-to-date emergency contact information for surrogate decision makers
- Making referrals for social services, ethics committees, or other resources to address conflicts related to healthcare decisions and interventions
- Teaching about interventions for comfort
- Providing information about palliative care
- Encouraging families and care partners to express their feelings and expressing compassion
- Suggesting referrals for caregiver support programs and other appropriate resources

========================*FAST FACTS in a NUTSHELL*

Nurses have many opportunities to simply communicate empathy for families and care partners who are dealing with challenging decisions about care of the person with advanced dementia.

## COMFORT FEEDING

Feeding and eating difficulties usually begin during the middle stage of dementia and gradually worsen. Major care issues in advanced dementia include increased risk for dehydration, weight loss, nutritional deficits, and aspiration pneumonia. Nurses, families, and care partners experience complex and powerful emotional and ethical concerns in addressing feeding and eating difficulties. Since the 1990s, percutaneous endoscopic gastrostomy (PEG) tubes have been used to provide fluid and nutrition to people with dementia. More recently, however, many questions have been raised about this practice because evidence does not support this intervention for people with advanced dementia. Current emphasis is on *comfort feeding only* as the best practice for addressing feeding and eating difficulties.

Because people with advanced dementia cannot participate in complex decision making, families and care partners need accurate information about interventions for nutrition, including the insertion of PEG tubes. Nurses can teach about the following points when they discuss this with families and care partners:

- There is no evidence supporting the use of feeding tubes as an effective intervention in people with advanced dementia.
- Feeding tubes are associated with complications (e.g., physical or pharmacological restraints and deprivation of the pleasure of food).
- Foregoing tube feeding does not mean the person's nutritional needs will be ignored.
- The intervention of *comfort feeding only* means that the person will not be forced to eat but will receive as much assistance as needed and will be fed so long as the process is not distressing.
- Comfort food is defined as any food that the person will accept, eat, and tolerate.
- Nursing and dietary staff will work with families and other care partners to identify the most appropriate and acceptable foods and fluids for the person with advanced dementia.
- Related interventions include providing meticulous oral care and using verbal and nonverbal communication that is comforting and encouraging during the feeding process.

In addition to talking with families about this issue, nurses are responsible for implementing these interventions, which can be very time consuming. In short-term care settings, if patient care assistants are available, nurses can teach them about comfort feeding techniques and allow enough time for hand feeding. Nurses may need to arrange for more flexible and frequent meal times for patients with advanced dementia and plan these around the availability of someone who can take time for the hand-feeding process. In addition, nurses in short-term care settings need to consider whether a referral for a dietary consultation or swallowing evaluation would be appropriate.

=*FAST FACTS in a NUTSHELL*

Care providers address complex and emotional issues related to usual care issues such as food and fluids.

🔅 **CLINICAL SNAPSHOT:** Mrs. V is admitted to the hospital with aspiration pneumonia. She resides in a nursing home and a swallowing evaluation indicates that she requires honey-thick foods. Mrs. V's daughter tells you that her mother does not like the thickened diet and she often finds cookies, crackers, and other snacks to eat in the drawers of other residents. You initiate referrals for a speech therapist and dietician to advise about foods that are safe and acceptable for Mrs. V.

## END-OF-LIFE CARE
## FOR ADVANCED DEMENTIA

A major challenge for families and care partners of people with advanced dementia is determining when the person moves into the terminal phase, which is generally defined as the 6 months prior to death. Of course, there is no crystal ball to predict the timeline, but the following factors are considered in determining hospice eligibility based on an expected 6-month survival:

- Progressive loss of all verbal and psychomotor abilities (Functional Assessment Staging 7)
- Dementia-related comorbidities: sepsis, aspiration, persistent fever, upper urinary tract infection, multiple stage 3–4 pressure ulcers, and significant weight loss within 6 months
- Significant comorbidities: cancer, congestive heart failure, unstable medical condition
- Additional considerations: oxygen therapy needed, shortness of breath, less than 25% of food eaten at most meals, bowel incontinence, sleeping most of the time

When dementia progresses to the terminal phase, goals increasingly focus on comfort and quality of life and there is less emphasis on curative interventions for concomitant conditions. Some treatment issues that often arise during this stage are:

- Discontinuing cholinesterase inhibitors
- Discontinuing memantine
- Discontinuing preventive medications (e.g., statins for cholesterol)
- Foregoing diagnostic procedures for nonacute symptoms
- Adhering to therapeutic diets
- Having the person evaluated in an emergency room or admitted to an acute care facility for non-life-threatening or nonpainful symptoms
- Initiating a referral for hospice services
- Discontinuing or initiating dialysis or tube feeding

When these decisions are being discussed or becoming imminent, nurses can suggest that a referral for hospice be considered. It is not necessary to know for certain that the person meets specific criteria because a hospice nurse or social worker will assess the situation and meet with designated decision makers to discuss services, determine eligibility, and advise the family.

## ═══════════════════════════════════ FAST FACTS in a NUTSHELL

Nurses can encourage families and designated decision makers to initiate a phone call to hospice programs to find out about this resource for people with advanced dementia.

## NURSING CARE FOR COMFORT

People with advanced dementia need physical and emotional comfort but they are unable to verbally express these needs. Interventions that nurses can incorporate in usual care activities include the following:

- Assume that the person understands the meaning of nonverbal communication and is aware of what you are communicating with body language
- Avoid being abrupt or hurried in verbal and nonverbal interactions
- Make a warm and personal connection with the person by smiling, touching gently, using a soft voice, and making eye contact
- Avoid terminology that is disrespectful
- Anticipate needs related to pain, discomfort, positioning, food, fluids, toileting, and level of physical activity
- Provide a therapeutic environment by controlling noise and lighting as much as possible (e.g., turn televisions to soothing music rather than to verbally intense programs)

## *FAST FACTS in a NUTSHELL*

Assume that people with advanced dementia understand verbal and nonverbal communication and communicate in a respectful and caring manner at all times.

## *RESOURCES in a NUTSHELL*

*Alzheimer's Association*

*www.alz.org*

*Hartford Institute for Geriatric Nursing*

*consultgerirn.org*

*National Hospice and Palliative Care Organization*

*nhpco.org*

# Issues Posing Particular Challenges in Clinical Settings

# 9

# Issues Related to Specific Care Settings

## INTRODUCTION

*Nurses who care for older adults in any health care setting are likely to care for patients who have dementia as a secondary diagnosis. It is not unusual or unprofessional to feel frustrated and unprepared and to view these situations as challenging and time consuming. Because the primary focus is on predominant medical problems, issues associated with a dementia diagnosis may be overlooked. It is important to recognize dementia-related issues to avoid a potentially frustrating situation; it may even be helpful to view dementia as a chronic condition similar to diabetes. From this perspective, both diabetes and dementia are chronic conditions that: (a) complicate the overall situation, (b) can be exacerbated during medical or surgical events, (c) require ongoing assessment, (d) require that additional interventions be incorporated into the usual care plan, and (e) present unique challenges and opportunities for providing person-centered care. A major difference is that nurses have guidelines for care of patients with diabetes but they are less likely to have clear guidelines related to the needs of people who have dementia. This chapter focuses on dementia-related issues that nurses commonly address when they work in specific care settings covered by health insurance. If you work in one of the settings discussed in this chapter, you can use the information to supplement all other chapters in this book.*

In this chapter, you will learn:

1. Nursing strategies to address dementia-related issues in emergency room settings
2. Nursing strategies to address dementia-related issues in acute care settings
3. Nursing strategies to address dementia-related issues in hospice programs
4. Nursing strategies to address dementia-related issues in skilled care settings

## ISSUES ASSOCIATED WITH EMERGENCY ROOM SETTINGS

Nurses in emergency rooms often care for a patient with dementia who arrives from a nursing facility for an evaluation of a change in mental status or for treatment of injuries sustained during a fall. These patients are likely to be accompanied only by the transporters, who present an envelope containing a list of diagnoses and medications and a brief overview of the reason for the patient being sent to the emergency room. The information is likely to report a "change in mental status" with little or no information about the person's usual level of functioning and baseline mental status. The arrival of such a patient presents several challenges.

## Establishing Accurate Patient Information

The initial challenge is to find out what the change entails and to assess for delirium, as discussed in Chapter 2. People with moderate and advanced dementia are particularly challenging because they are likely to report something totally unrelated to or different from the reported presenting problem. For example, they may not be able to verbally describe their symptoms or they may use words that do not accurately describe the location of pain. In addition, the person's mental status is likely to be compromised by the confusion of being in an unfamiliar environment. In these situations, the assessment of the reason for the emergency evaluation may differ significantly from the information received from the referring facility.

A related issue is that information about current medications may be incomplete or inaccurate, so it is difficult to know how medications are affecting the person's condition. If the person has a list of medications, it may be outdated or not include recently prescribed or "as needed" medications. Also, it may not include over-the-counter medications, which can be a contributing factor in the change in condition. In all these situations, it is necessary to obtain as much information as possible from the person with dementia and then confirm the accuracy of this information with someone who can verify or amplify the information.

=====*FAST FACTS in a NUTSHELL*

Check for nonprescription medications that can affect mental status. For example, many people take diphenhydramine (Benadryl) as a sleep aid and do not recognize that this can cause cognitive impairment, especially in older adults.

Some strategies for obtaining assessment information when caring for someone with dementia include:

- Check for any form of identification (i.e., medic alert bracelet, necklace, or wallet card) that includes a toll-free number to call for medical history and information about contact people. When you call the toll-free number, ask how recently this information was updated.
- Contact the person's care partners and request information.
- Call the nursing facility and talk with the usual nurse on the unit from which the patient was sent; ask for baseline functioning and mental status, current medications, detailed description of the change, and reason for being sent.
- Ask care partners to bring all containers from currently and recently used medications, including nonprescription products.
- Call the person's pharmacy to obtain information about current and recently prescribed medications.
- Review any medical record available in your facility.
- Fax or call for a release of information form requesting medical records from the physician's office or another health care facility.

## Managing Behavioral Manifestations

Another nursing challenge associated with caring for people with dementia in emergency rooms is addressing common behavioral manifestations, such as agitation and increased confusion. An important intervention is to find someone to stay with the person—but this is not always easy. When hospital social workers are not available to assist, emergency room nurses may need to assume this responsibility. Nurses can try the following ways of finding a companion for people with dementia:

- Look for contact information on the person's chart or ask the person with dementia if there is someone you can call to come.
- If the person with dementia was sent from a nursing or assisted living facility, you can call and ask that an aide, companion, or any other contact person come to the emergency room.
- Some hospitals provide sitter or companion services or have a list of agencies that families can contact to arrange for these services, and emergency room nurses can initiate a referral as an intervention for patient safety.

### Detecting Elder Abuse

Another issue is that emergency room nurses need to be on alert not only for obvious manifestations of elder abuse (e.g., bruises, suspicious injuries) but also for subtle signs of abuse or self-neglect (e.g., malnutrition, medication mismanagement, and alcohol abuse). Additional nursing considerations related to detection of elder abuse are:

- If there are concerns about malnutrition, suggest that the person be evaluated by obtaining a serum albumin level.
- If the person with dementia is brought to an emergency room because he or she is lost and cannot find the way home, consider that this can be a form of elder neglect.
- Whenever there is evidence of elder abuse or neglect, there is an obligation to follow the hospital protocol with regard to reporting and follow-up, as described in Chapter 15.

## ACUTE CARE SETTINGS

Older adults with dementia are more likely than those without this diagnosis to be admitted to a hospital and are more likely to stay longer for management of coexisting conditions such as diabetes, cancer, and heart disease (Alzheimer's Association, 2009). A study of community-dwelling older adults with dementia identified the leading causes for hospital admission as syncope or falls, ischemic heart disease, gastrointestinal disorders, pneumonia, and delirium (Rudolph et al., 2010). A review of studies concluded that at least one third of people with dementia are hospitalized each year, and about one fourth of older patients in hospital settings have dementia (Maslow, 2006).

Even though dementia is a common diagnosis, it will not necessarily be documented on the patient's chart if it is not the primary reason for the admission. Also, because dementia develops gradually and can be exacerbated by a medical condition or disruption in the person's routine, the hospitalization itself may become the "straw that breaks the camel's back" that raises questions about dementia as a probable diagnosis. In these situations, nurses may need to address issues related to diagnosing dementia, as discussed in Chapter 6. If you suspect that a patient has undiagnosed dementia, you can use the family questionnaire or patient behavior assessment tool listed in the Resources in a Nutshell section at the end of this chapter.

## Programs That Provide Dementia Patient Guidelines in Acute Care

In recent years, many hospitals have initiated programs to address the unique needs of patients with dementia, and nurses need to be aware of any available resources within their institutions. Two outstanding initiatives that are widely available in hospitals throughout the United States are Acute Care for the Elderly (ACE) units and the Nurses Improving

Care for the Hospitalized Elderly (NICHE) program of the Hartford Institute for Geriatric Nursing.

- ACE units are designated hospital units that provide a multidisciplinary approach to preventing and managing complex geriatric syndromes. If you work in a hospital that has an ACE unit, you can ask for a consultation about care of patients with dementia, including consideration that the patient be transferred to that unit.
- The NICHE program encourages the development of the Geriatric Resource Nurse model so a specially trained geriatric nurse is available to work with staff nurses. If you work in a NICHE hospital, you can request advice from one of these nurses to assist with development of appropriate care plans for patients with dementia.

Nurses who do not have access to specialized resources or programs can suggest referrals for assessment and interventions to appropriate professional colleagues, including:

- Geriatric clinical nurse specialist or geriatric resource nurse for assistance and consultation related to care planning
- Geropsychiatrist, neurologist, or geriatrician for evaluation of mental status and recommendations about management
- Social worker for discussions with care partners and assistance with discharge planning
- Social worker for information about helpful community services, such as the Alzheimer's Association
- Speech therapist for cognitive therapies
- Occupational therapist for safety and independence in activities of daily living (including driving rehabilitation)

- Physical therapist for maintaining safe mobility and preventing falls and excess disability
- Speech therapist for assessment and recommendations related to chewing, swallowing, and safe eating
- Pastoral care for assistance with spiritual care

## Managing Behavioral Manifestations

Another common issue for nurses in acute care settings is managing daily care activities and behavioral manifestations for patients with dementia. In addition to the interventions discussed in Chapters 10 through 14 in this book, it is important to obtain information about effective interventions that were used by care partners before the patient was hospitalized. This information can be obtained by talking with the patient's care partners when they visit and by calling nursing staff or family members who provided care in the home or long-term care settings. It also is imperative that this information is incorporated into the written care plan and that pertinent and effective strategies are communicated during shift reports. This is especially important for patients with moderate or advanced dementia who cannot communicate about their needs.

## HOSPICE PROGRAMS

When hospice care—which provides services across all health care settings—was established in the United States in the 1970s, a diagnosis of cancer was the predominant reason for admission and advanced dementia was not a covered diagnosis. In 2009, cancer was the primary diagnosis for only about 40% of hospice recipients and dementia was the primary diagnosis for 11.2% (National Hospice and Palliative

Care Organization, 2010). Because an additional 19% of hospice recipients have a secondary diagnosis of dementia, the diagnosis of dementia is more common in hospice settings than in hospitals (Legler, Bradley, & Carlson, 2011; Torke et al., 2010). Overall, about 29% of people receiving hospice care have dementia.

## Identifying and Establishing Dementia Patient Guidelines in Hospice Programs

Although all hospice programs have guidelines for patients admitted with a primary diagnosis of advanced dementia, they do not have guidelines for patients who have dementia as a secondary diagnosis or for patients in early and moderate stages. Some hospice programs have specialized dementia services, but most of these focus on issues related to advanced dementia. If a hospice program has not yet developed specialized services for care of people with dementia, useful information can be accessed on the National Hospice and Palliative Care Organization website (nhpco.org) in the section on professional resources/access.

## Developing Person-Centered Care Within the Health Care Team

Hospice patients with dementia present many challenges related to assessment, communication, decisions regarding treatment, and the needs of family and other care partners. Because hospice programs are interdisciplinary, nurses have the advantage of addressing these complex issues as part of a health care team. In the team context, nurses assume primary responsibility for assessment and management of pain and comfort, as discussed in Chapter 10. Nurses can apply information from all chapters of this book to assist the team in developing a person-centered care plan that addresses dementia-related issues.

═══════════════════════════════════*FAST FACTS in a NUTSHELL*

🌀 **CLINICAL SNAPSHOT:** Mrs. H is admitted for hospice care because of metastasis from breast cancer but she has a secondary diagnosis of dementia. The hospice nurse obtains information from the Alzheimer's Association about tips for care of people with dementia and discusses this during a clinical conference with the hospice team.

## SKILLED CARE SETTINGS

Nurses provide skilled care services in homes, residential facilities, and nursing and rehabilitation facilities. Skilled nursing care is defined as medically necessary services for people who require daily or intermittent care provided by a registered nurse in a Medicare-certified facility or by a Medicare-certified home care agency. Because skilled nursing services are short term based on strict qualifications, continuity of care is a common issue. This is particularly problematic for people with dementia because they require more time and support to reach skilled care goals and they are likely to become disqualified for care before they or their care partners think they are ready for discharge. For example, many older adults require skilled care when they are discharged from acute care settings, but they receive only an average of about 23 days of Medicare-covered service because they do not meet the criteria for the full 100 days that might be covered.

## Optimizing Skilled Care Services and Continuity of Care

Because of the short-term nature of skilled care and the complexity of patient needs, nurses providing skilled care services to dementia patients in home or institutional settings need to be proactive in planning for the next level of care.

- One approach is to initiate a timely referral for medical social work services that are available as part of skilled care. This is especially important because many of the services that are necessary when people no longer qualify for skilled care are not covered by health insurance. Some services, however, may be covered by long-term care insurance for the small percentage of people who have purchased those policies.
- Nurses also can suggest referrals for the types of services that are available to address needs of people with dementia and their care partners, as discussed in Chapter 16.

═══════════════════════════════════*FAST FACTS in a NUTSHELL*

Because skilled nursing services are short term and the needs of patients with dementia are complex, nurses need to be proactive in planning continuity of care.

🔲 **CLINICAL SNAPSHOT:** Ms. B was admitted for skilled therapy after surgery for a total hip replacement. Her daughter assumed she would be in the facility for several weeks, but Ms. B qualifies for only 9 days of therapy because she has moderate dementia and has not been able to learn how to use her walker without assistance. You suggest that Ms. B's daughter begin exploring options for care at home and you ask the social worker to provide information.

## ═══════════RESOURCES in a NUTSHELL

### Alzheimer's Association

*www.alz.org*

- Information to assist care partners in preparing for hospitalization of a person with dementia

### Hartford Institute for Geriatric Nursing

*consultgerirn.org/resources*

- Recognition of Dementia in Hospitalized Older Adults, *Try This*, Issue D5, and video demonstrating application of the assessment tool
- Working With Families of Hospitalized Older Adults With Dementia, *Try This*, Issue D10, and video demonstrating application of the assessment tool

### National Hospice and Palliative Care Organization

*www.nhpco.org*

- Guidelines for hospice services for persons with dementia

### Article

The Special Needs of the Hospitalized Patient With Dementia by T. Weitzel, S. Robinson, M. R. Barnes, T. A. Berry, J. M. Holmes, S. Mercer, . . . G. L. Kirkbride, *Medsurg Nursing*, January-February 2011, Vol. 20, No. 1, pp. 13–18.

# 10

## Assessing and Managing Pain

### INTRODUCTION

*In recent years, there is increasing attention to the experience and management of pain in people with dementia. Current conclusions are that people with dementia:*

- *Are likely to experience pain at a higher rate than those who are cognitively intact*
- *Are less likely to have it treated adequately*
- *Are less likely to self-report and seek relief*
- *Are able to communicate verbally about pain during mild and moderate stages, but it may be difficult to decipher their messages*
- *Communicate in nonverbal ways, including through emotions and behaviors, during advanced dementia*

*In an effort to address these concerns, dementia experts have identified assessment methods and management protocols that nurses can use when they care for people with dementia.*

In this chapter, you will learn:

1. How to assess for pain in people with dementia
2. Effective ways of managing pain in people with dementia

## ASSESSING PAIN IN PEOPLE WITH DEMENTIA

Pain assessment in people with dementia is challenging, especially when there is a combination of acute and chronic conditions or when nurses do not know the person's usual ways of communicating about pain. When caring for people with mild or moderate dementia, nurses can try the following techniques to elicit information about the person's experience of pain:

• Ask the person what words they usually use when they talk about pain.
• Offer examples of words that communicate pain and discomfort: hurting, sore, achy, tender, and ouch.
• Ask "Are you hurting or uncomfortable in any way?"
• If you suspect that an area is painful or uncomfortable, point or use gentle touch, and ask "How does your _____ [knee, head, stomach] feel now?"
• When people with dementia report pain or discomfort in a specific area, ask them to point to the area to verify the location (e.g., they may say their head hurts, but point to their shoulder when asked to verify).

In addition, nurses can obtain information from the person's family and care partners by asking if there are particular words or ways the person typically uses to communicate about pain or discomfort.

As the ability to self-report about experiences of pain diminishes during the course of dementia, nurses and care partners increasingly rely on observations and other sources of information to assess pain in people with moderate and advanced dementia. For instance, nurses can review the patient's chart for information about chronic or recurring conditions that are associated with pain and are likely to be undertreated. Examples include arthritis, fibromyalgia, back pain, postherpetic neuralgia, and diabetic neuropathies. Nurses have many opportunities to observe indicators of pain or discomfort and document these as an integral aspect of pain assessment. Table 10.1 lists indicators and examples that serve as "red flags" for the presence of pain or discomfort, particularly in people with advanced dementia.

### TABLE 10.1  Indicators of Pain or Discomfort

| Indicator | Examples |
| --- | --- |
| Recent falls or other injuries that can cause pain | Bruises, burns, wounds, skin tears |
| Recent or potentially recurrent infections or other conditions | Urinary tract infections, constipation, fecal impaction |
| Physical changes | Redness, swelling, elevated temperature |
| Verbalizations or vocalizations | Moans, groans, cries, whimpering |
| Movement of arms and legs | Guarding, diminished weight-bearing ability, limited range of motion |
| Overall movements | Restlessness, shifting positions, repetitive hand movements, rubbing or massaging affected area |
| Response during activities or treatments | Resistance, protective actions, tightening, combativeness |
| Behaviors | Agitation, irritability, increased confusion, change in mental status |
| Activities of daily living | Poor appetite, increased dependency, changes in functioning |
| Psychosocial function | Mood swings, withdrawal from usual social activities, agitation, changes in relationships |

━━━━━━━━━━━━━━━━━━━━━━*FAST FACTS in a NUTSHELL*

People with dementia do communicate about pain, but they may do so indirectly, nonverbally, or verbally but imprecisely.

💠 **CLINICAL SNAPSHOT:** Mrs. E is admitted to the hospital for management of congestive heart failure, and she also has moderate dementia. When you provide standby assistance for walking to the bathroom, she grabs your arm for more assistance and you note that she does not bear full weight on her left leg. You ask if her leg hurts, and she says, "Oh, it's OK but I think I stubbed my finger." You assess her lower extremities and observe that her left big toe is red and swollen. She is diagnosed with gout, which has been exacerbated by the physiologic stress of her medical condition.

## Using Pain-Rating Scales

Pain, which is viewed as the "fourth vital sign," is assessed according to universally recognized scales, such as "on a scale of 1 to 10, with 10 being the most severe level. . . ." People with mild and moderate dementia usually maintain some ability to self-report and respond to a simple verbal scale such as those commonly in use. However, if they have difficulty processing information, their responses may not be accurate; and even if the response is accurate, a rating scale is only one small piece of information about the person's experience of pain, particularly for people with dementia. Thus, nurses need to supplement information from the pain scales by assessing the indicators listed in Table 10.1.

The Pain Assessment in Advanced Dementia (PAIN-AD), the Checklist of Nonverbal Pain Indicators (CNPI), and the Pain Assessment Checklist for Seniors with Limited Ability to Communicate (PACSLAC) are examples of rating scales that nurses can use to assess pain in people with advanced dementia. The Resources in a Nutshell section at the end of this chapter lists Internet sites for information about these and other tools that document assessment observations. A precaution for nurses in short-term care settings is that some tools require observations of changes over time.

=====*FAST FACTS in a NUTSHELL*

When assessing pain in people who cannot reliably self-report, nurses supplement information on standard pain assessment tools with assessment observations as detailed in Table 10.1.

**CLINICAL SNAPSHOT:** When nurses ask Mr. G to rate his pain on a scale of 1 to 10, he always responds with "10, 10, 10, I told you already." Because he has a secondary diagnosis of dementia, nurses document that he "shows no signs of discomfort or pain and has no areas of redness or swelling, but moans and tightens his arms when he is transferred to the bedside commode with 2-person assist."

## MANAGING PAIN IN PEOPLE WITH DEMENTIA

As with all patient care situations, nurses work closely with physicians and other team members to implement appropriate measures for treatment of pain and medical conditions. This approach involves pharmacologic and nonpharmacologic interventions and ongoing assessment of effectiveness and adverse effects of medications. In addition, when caring for people with dementia, it is important to recognize that expressions of pain or discomfort, especially during moderate or advanced stages, are often due to simple unmet needs such as:

• Feeling hungry or thirsty
• Feeling too hot or too cold
• Lying or sitting in wet or soiled bedding or clothing
• Needing assistance with activities of daily living (e.g., toileting)

- Unavailability of assistive devices (e.g., mobility aids, clean eyeglasses)
- Hearing aids ringing in their ears or being out of place
- Feeling emotional discomfort (e.g., sad, lonely, bored)
- Experiencing their environment as too noisy or over-stimulating

Thus, an important nursing intervention is to identify and address basic physical and emotional needs as much as possible.

Dementia experts increasingly emphasize that unrecognized and untreated pain due to chronic conditions (referred to as *persistent pain*) is a common cause of discomfort and challenging behaviors. The connection between pain and behavior may not be obvious, especially when the pain is due to long-term conditions and the person with dementia has limited verbal abilities. Nurses can apply all the assessment guidelines discussed previously in this chapter, and then determine whether chronic pain is potentially a cause of challenging behaviors or whether it affects functioning or quality of life for the person with dementia. If there is reason to suspect the person is experiencing pain or discomfort from a chronic condition that is medically controlled as much as possible, a trial of analgesic medications may be warranted. Studies have found that effective pain management can reduce agitation and other behaviors in people with moderate and advanced dementia (Husebo, Ballard, Sandvik, Nilsen, & Aarsland, 2011).

## Pharmacologic Management of Pain

Highlights of evidence-based guidelines for pharmacologic management of persistent pain in older adults published by the American Geriatrics Society (2009) are as follows:

- Analgesics should be initiated at low doses and titrated upward for optimum pain relief and minimal adverse effects.
- Initial and ongoing evaluation of therapeutic and adverse effects is essential.

- Regular, rather than as needed, doses are preferable for people who are cognitively impaired and cannot request medications appropriately.
- Medications should be provided around the clock for people with continuous pain.
- A combination of medications with complementary actions may work synergistically for better relief and less toxicity than higher doses of a single agent.
- Pharmacologic interventions should be combined with nonpharmacologic approaches to enhance effectiveness.

Table 10.2 summarizes guidelines for pharmacologic management of persistent pain in older adults.

**TABLE 10.2  Guidelines for Pharmacologic Management of Persistent Pain in Older Adults**

| Medication | Indications and Maximum Dose |
| --- | --- |
| Acetaminophen (Tylenol) for musculoskeletal conditions (e.g., osteoarthritis and low back pain) | 650–1,000 mg every 6–8 hours; lower dose with hepatic insufficiency or history of alcohol abuse; lower dose if combined with opioids |
| Nonsteroidal anti-inflammatory drugs (NSAIDs) for chronic inflammatory conditions (e.g., rheumatoid arthritis) or short-term relief of musculoskeletal conditions | Caution with renal insufficiency, gastropathy, hypertension, cardiovascular disease, and congestive heart failure; avoid coadministration with low-dose aspirin |
| Opioid analgesics if nonopioids are ineffective or if significant risk of serious adverse effects from NSAIDs or acetaminophen; effective for neuropathic pain conditions (diabetic neuropathy, postherpetic neuralgia) | Begin trial basis with clearly defined goals and discontinue if goals are not achieved; assess, prevent, and treat constipation |
| Adjuvant drugs such as antidepressants, anticonvulsants (e.g., gabapentin [Neurontin], pregabalin [Lyrica]) | Used alone or in combination with analgesics for certain conditions (e.g., fibromyalgia, neuropathic pain); evaluate anticholinergic or sedating adverse effects |

*(continued)*

**TABLE 10.2  Guidelines for Pharmacologic Management of Persistent Pain in Older Adults** *(continued)*

| Medication | Indications and Maximum Dose |
|---|---|
| Corticosteroids for rheumatic and autoimmune conditions (rheumatoid arthritis, giant cell arteritis) | Use lowest dose for the shortest time; evaluate, prevent, and manage adverse effects of long-term administration (e.g., interventions to prevent osteoporotic fractures) |
| Lidocaine patch (Fentanyl) for neuropathic pain | Adverse reactions are rare, mild, and mostly related to local skin irritation; contraindicated in advanced liver failure |
| Topical capsaicin cream (Capzasin) | Common adverse effect of burning sensation, which may persist for several months |
| Topical NSAIDs (e.g., aspirin, indomethacin [Indocin], diclofenac [Voltaren], piroxicam [Feldene], ketoprofen [Actron]) | Minimal adverse effects due to low systemic absorption |

=====================≡*FAST FACTS in a NUTSHELL*

Agitation in people with moderate or advanced dementia may be caused by persistent pain.

🌀 **CLINICAL SNAPSHOT:** Mr. P has advanced dementia and has a history of arthritis in both knees and hips. He rarely gets out of the chair, even though he has good mobility and balance. When nursing assistants encourage him to walk to the dining room, he becomes combative and yells, "No, no!" After he begins taking acetaminophen 750 mg every 6 hours, he is less agitated and willing to walk several times a day.

## Nonpharmacologic Interventions

Many nonpharmacologic interventions are effective for persistent pain and these may be particularly helpful for people with mild or moderate dementia. Nurses can suggest the following interventions that can enhance pain management:

- Yoga
- Reiki
- Aquatherapy
- Massage
- Therapeutic touch
- Acupuncture
- Meditation
- Visual or auditory distraction (calming music, scenes of nature)

Nurses can suggest a referral for physical therapy for pain management interventions that might be covered by health insurance. Nurses also can suggest that community centers and health centers offer resources for many of these interventions, which sometimes are covered by insurance or provided at a discounted rate.

═══════════════════════════════*FAST FACTS in a NUTSHELL*

Nurses have many opportunities to suggest nonpharmacologic interventions for persistent pain in people with dementia, such as physical therapy for musculoskeletal conditions. People with mild dementia are capable of engaging in self-care activities such as yoga or meditation.

🌀 **CLINICAL SNAPSHOT:** Mr. R, who has mild dementia, is being discharged from rehabilitation following recovery

*(continued)*

(*continued*)

from total hip replacement surgery. His wife asks if there are other things he can do to address his discomfort and maintain his walking and balance. You suggest they both consider joining the weekly tai chi classes that are held at the senior center where they have gone for meals.

# RESOURCES in a NUTSHELL

*American Geriatrics Society, Foundation for Health in Aging*

*www.healthinaging.org*

• Pain in Dementia: Family and Caregivers Guide to Assessment and Treatment

*Geriatric Pain*

*www.geriatricpain.org*

*Hartford Institute for Geriatric Nursing*

*www.consultgerirn.org*

• Assessing Pain in Persons with Dementia, *Try This*, Issue D2, and video illustrating application of assessment tool
• Using Pain-Rating Scales in Older Adults, *Try This*, Issue 7, and video illustrating application of assessment tools
• Assessment of Nociceptive Versus Neuropathic Pain in Older Adults, *Try This*, Issue SP1

# II

# Addressing Safety Issues:
# Falls, Restraints, and Wandering

## INTRODUCTION

*Nurses caring for people with dementia frequently address safety issues, including falls and unsafe wandering. Safety concerns are usually heightened when people with dementia are in unfamiliar environments and when they have medical problems. Although physical restraints have been used in the past, health care professionals now recognize that restraints are rarely an appropriate intervention for ensuring safety. Nurses need to address safety issues as an important aspect of care for people with dementia.*

In this chapter, you will learn:

1. How to assess fall risks in people with dementia
2. Interventions for preventing falls and fall-related injuries
3. How to avoid the use of restraints
4. How to address wandering

# PREVENTING FALLS IN PEOPLE WITH DEMENTIA

People with dementia are at high risk for falls, and half of the falls in people with dementia result in injury, including hip fractures. Falls usually are attributed to a combination of risk conditions, which tend to be cumulative as dementia progresses. Nursing responsibilities include identifying and addressing conditions that increase the risk for falls or fall-related injuries.

## Assessing Fall Risk

Institutional settings routinely incorporate fall risk assessment tools as an integral part of the nursing assessment, but it is important to recognize that these tools are not specifically for people with dementia. Nurses need to add another layer to their fall risk assessment and consider conditions that increase the risk for falls in people with dementia. Goin, Duke, Hollawell, Horton, and Voytek (2011) have identified the following risks in people with moderate and advanced dementia:

*General Considerations*
- New admission or transfer
- Fall(s) within past month
- Bladder and/or bowel incontinence
- Seizures
- Acute illness

*Cognitive Factors*
- Depression
- Impaired judgment

- Unable to recognize ambulation deficits
- Unable to verbally communicate needs

### Sensory Function
- Decreased depth perception
- Decreased peripheral vision
- Unable to tolerate wearing eyeglasses or hearing aids

### Gait, Balance, and Mobility Factors
- Ambulatory but weak or debilitated
- Unable to use assistive devices properly
- Impaired balance
- Altered gait: shuffling, hesitancy, slow, unsteady, postural sway

### Neuromotor Function
- Rigidity of neck, torso, extremities
- Decreased grip strength
- Poor protective reflexes

### Behaviors
- Wandering
- Restless pacing
- Resistance to care
- Anxiety, agitation
- Sleep disturbances

Nurses assess and document fall risks during the initial assessment and whenever the person's condition changes. This is especially important when caring for people whose mental status fluctuates, as is often the case with dementia.

════════════════════════════════════*FAST FACTS in a NUTSHELL*

When caring for people with dementia, nurses need to supplement standard assessment tools and document additional dementia-specific risks.

## Addressing Fall Risks

Although it may be easy to fill out a fall risk checklist and place it in a patient's chart, the difficult—but essential—nursing responsibility is to address all the conditions that are amenable to interventions. Table 11.1 describes potentially reversible risk conditions and associated nursing actions to address these common risks. An additional consideration is that nurses need to take more initiative and be proactive when caring for people who are cognitively compromised, as at all levels of dementia. For example, it may be appropriate to request full-time assistance provided by family, care partners (if appropriate), or paid companions (if available).

════════════════════════════════════*FAST FACTS in a NUTSHELL*

Nurses have many opportunities to address conditions that are identified in fall risk assessment tools.

🔘 CLINICAL SNAPSHOT: Mr. W is admitted with a primary diagnosis of aspiration pneumonia and secondary diagnoses of Parkinson's disease and advanced dementia. He usually walks with a walker and one assist, but he has fallen several times during the past 6 months. He is very confused and frequently attempts to get out of bed. Family members tell you they can take turns staying at his bedside during the day, but they are unable to do so at night. You ask for orders for physical therapy and a social service consult to talk with the family about a bedside companion to fill the hours when he will be unattended.

## TABLE 11.1  Nursing Actions to Address Fall Risks

| Risk Condition | Nursing Actions |
|---|---|
| Poor balance, impaired mobility, bed rest, muscular weakness | Assist as necessary to maintain maximum level of safe mobility.<br>Request physical therapy for evaluation and treatment.<br>Provide range of motion exercise at least daily as appropriate.<br>Teach family and care partners about assisting with exercise and safe mobility.<br>For people being discharged to community settings: Consider referral for physical therapy follow-up through home care agency for homebound people and in outpatient setting for people who are not homebound. |
| Adverse medication effects | Talk with prescribing practitioners about anticholinergics and other medications that are associated with increased fall risk.<br>Obtain pharmacy consult to review and advise about medications. |
| Unable to request help or use call system | Assign room near nursing station.<br>Anticipate needs frequently, especially for toileting.<br>Make sure all staff know that the person is unable to ask for help.<br>Observe for nonverbal indicators of need and offer help.<br>Arrange for bedside companion to observe, assist, and call for help.<br>Use monitoring devices, such as pressure-activated pads with sound signals, and make sure that all staff are aware of the need to respond quickly to alerting devices. |
| Lack of sturdy nonslip footwear | Make sure the person uses nonskid foot protectors or appropriate shoes or slippers during transfers and ambulation. |
| Unsafe bedside environment | Assess bedside environment for items that contribute to falls (including walkers, wheelchairs, and medical equipment) and move any items that pose risks for falls or injury. |

*(continued)*

**TABLE 11.1  Nursing Actions to Address Fall Risks (*continued*)**

| Risk Condition | Nursing Actions |
| --- | --- |
| Inadequate physical activity | Discharge instructions: Teach about importance of engaging in safe and enjoyable physical activities (e.g., mall walking, video or television programs, and games).<br>Discharge instructions: Encourage participation in group activities for exercise (e.g., dancing, tai chi, walking clubs, Wii bowling, and other video-based programs). |
| Reduced vision | Make sure eyeglasses are clean and available and provide reminders or assistance if needed. |
| Unsafe home environment | Teach about a safe home environment: uncluttered, good lighting, no throw rugs, and no cords or other objects associated with tripping.<br>Teach about bathroom safety equipment: grab bars, elevated toilet seat, and tub seat or shower chair.<br>Consider referral for home evaluation by physical and occupational therapists as part of discharge plan for patients returning to home or community settings. |

## Preventing Fall-Related Injuries

In addition to taking action to prevent falls, nurses are responsible for implementing interventions to reduce fractures and other injuries when falls do occur. For example, nurses can address osteoporosis—which occurs to some degree in all men and women by age 75 and increases the risk of fractures—through interventions such as:

- Finding out if the person has had screening tests such as bone mineral density to evaluate for osteoporosis
- Encouraging discussion with the primary care provider about medications for osteoporosis if the person has a history of fractures
- Teaching about the importance of weight-bearing exercise for 30 minutes daily

- Teaching about adequate amounts of calcium (1,200–1,500 mg/day) and vitamin D (800–1,000 IU/day) in food or supplements

Another focus of nursing interventions is addressing environmental conditions that can cause cuts, bruises, bleeding, and other fall-related injuries. Examples of these interventions are:

- Keeping the bed in the lowest position
- Removing objects and furniture that can cause harm
- Keeping the environment uncluttered and safe
- Providing good lighting

===================================*FAST FACTS in a NUTSHELL*

Nurses can incorporate information about interventions for osteoporosis as a health promotion intervention for prevention of fractures.

**CLINICAL SNAPSHOT:** Mrs. O is 81 years old and is in the emergency room for evaluation of injuries sustained when she tripped at home. X-rays indicate she has no fractures, but she has a history of a fractured wrist 5 years ago. You encourage her to ask her doctor about osteoporosis and you teach her about a safe home environment.

## PHYSICAL RESTRAINTS

The Centers for Medicare and Medicaid defines a physical restraint as any manual method, physical or mechanical device, or equipment that is used to limit a person's movement of body, head, or extremities freely. Examples include hand mitts; elbow splints; full side rails; chairs with tabletops; and waist, vest, wrist, or leg restraints. Despite the common perception that physical restraints protect from falls, there is little evidence of effectiveness and much evidence of detrimental effects. Poor outcomes associated with physical restraints in people with dementia include:

- Exacerbation of confusion
- Increased agitation and anxiety
- Increased risk of fall-related injury
- Negative emotional responses, including fear, anger, resistance, and humiliation
- Physical deconditioning
- Decline in functioning
- Bruises, skin tears, pressure ulcers
- Urinary incontinence
- Constipation and fecal impaction
- Musculoskeletal injury (strains, contractures, limited range of motion)
- Strangulation or asphyxiation

## Avoiding Restraints

A combination of evidence-based information about adverse effects of physical restraints and the increasing focus on person-centered care for people with dementia has led to the development of "restraint-free" care in institutional settings. Interventions for avoiding restraints include all those discussed for fall prevention (Table 11.1) and interventions to address dementia-associated behaviors, as discussed in Chapter 13. Interventions related to invasive treatment devices include:

- Using the least invasive method to deliver care
- Repeatedly communicating about the purpose of the treatment in terms the person can understand
- Protecting and camouflaging the device with clothing, protective sleeve, or temporary air splint

- Soliciting assistance from family, care partners, and activities staff to provide diversionary activities
- Discontinuing invasive treatments as soon as possible

================ *FAST FACTS in a NUTSHELL*

Physical restraints are not effective for reducing falls and they are associated with many adverse effects, including increased risk for fall-related injuries.

## WANDERING AND PACING

One of the major reasons for consideration of restraints is that people with dementia often exhibit wandering or pacing. Even though these behaviors may appear to be purposeless, people with dementia may be looking for ways to meet their physical or emotional needs. Wandering and pacing also may be indicators of motor restlessness associated with adverse medication effects or medical conditions. Any of the following conditions can trigger wandering and pacing in a person with dementia:

- Physical discomfort (pain, hunger, thirst, or too hot or too cold)
- Physical need (finding a toilet)
- Need to change position (attempt at comfort or pain relief)
- Restlessness as adverse effect of medications (*akathisia*—severe motor restlessness due to antipsychotics or antidepressants—may look like persistent anxiety or aggressiveness)
- Stimulating effect of some drugs (caffeine, antidepressants)
- Anticholinergics can cause general feeling of restlessness
- Drugs may cause increased urge to urinate or defecate and may cause pacing
- Bowel or bladder disorders (UTI, constipation) may lead to pacing

- Medical conditions that can cause pacing and restlessness: depression, neuropathies, skin disorders, thyroid disease
- Dementia itself, depending on area of brain
- Overstimulation or understimulation (boredom)
- Believing they are elsewhere and need to do something (go to work, pick children up from school)
- Lack of exercise, need for physical activity
- Delayed reaction to overstimulation from the evening or day before

## Addressing Wandering and Pacing

Nurses can address conditions that trigger wandering and pacing by applying the interventions discussed in Chapter 13 for dementia-associated behaviors. Additional interventions, specific to addressing wandering and pacing in hospital settings, include:

- Providing appropriate supervision (e.g., placing in room that allows for maximum observation, frequently checking, and requesting assistance of companions or specialized staff)
- Using movement detection devices to alert staff (e.g., pressure pads with audible signal)
- Reducing environmental triggers (avoiding rooms near high levels of activity, keeping the person's street clothing and shoes out of sight)
- Providing orientation cues and frequent reminders (e.g., "You'll be staying in the hospital until you are better")
- Distracting the person's attention

========================*FAST FACTS in a NUTSHELL*

Nurses need to identify conditions and needs that trigger wandering and pacing and recognize that the behaviors are an attempt to meet a physical or emotional need.

# ═══════════════RESOURCES in a NUTSHELL

*Alzheimer's Association*

*www.alz.org*

- Reports and recommendations on falls, wandering, and physical restraints

*American Geriatrics Society, Clinical Practice Guideline on Prevention of Falls in Older Persons*

*www.americangeriatrics.org*

*Hartford Institute for Geriatric Nursing*

*www.consultgerirn.org*

- Fall Risk Assessment, *Try This*, Issue 5, and video illustrating application of assessment tool
- Avoiding Restraints in Older Adults with Dementia, *Try This*, Issue D1, article and video
- Wandering in Hospitalized Older Adults, *Try This*, Issue D6, article and video
- Evidence-based guidelines on use of physical restraints with elderly patients
- Nursing standards of practice protocol: Fall prevention

# 12

# Communicating With People Who Have Dementia

## INTRODUCTION

*Dementia affects verbal and nonverbal communication skills, and the effects of dementia progress throughout the course. Nurses need to assess communication difficulties and identify effective ways of communicating verbally and nonverbally. In fact, appropriate communication techniques are a major nursing intervention when caring for people with dementia.*

In this chapter, you will learn:

1. Communication issues associated with stages of dementia
2. Ways of improving verbal communication when caring for people with dementia
3. How to communicate respectfully
4. Effective ways of communicating nonverbally

## COMMUNICATION ISSUES ASSOCIATED WITH DEMENTIA

### Common Issues Occurring With Mild Dementia

Verbal communication is usually one of the first aspects of functioning that is affected by dementia-related brain changes; in some cases, verbal abilities are affected months or even years before memory deficits are noted. As dementia progresses, the person's ability to communicate verbally (i.e., expressive abilities) diminishes gradually; it eventually becomes severely compromised during the advanced stage. Similarly, one's ability to understand verbal communication (i.e., receptive abilities) also diminishes gradually. However, expressive and receptive abilities might not diminish at the same rate. Although people with mild dementia may be able to understand verbal communication, they may have difficulty expressing themselves, which can manifest through:

- Mispronunciation
- Incorrect grammar
- Inaccurate use of words
- Inability to finish sentences
- Inability to find the right word ("it's on the tip of my tongue but it can't come out")
- Using a general word when asked to name an item ("thing" instead of "pen")
- Difficulty following complex discussions
- Difficulty following conversations that are not one-on-one
- Difficulty communicating when the environment is noisy or otherwise distracting

In these situations, people with dementia and their families and care partners may benefit from speech therapy services so they can learn about techniques to facilitate communication. This is an aspect of care that often is overlooked, even though people with mild or moderate dementia can learn about techniques to improve communication. This is particularly important for people with dementia who have families and care partners who are interested in learning how to facilitate communication between themselves and the person with dementia.

═══════════════════════════════════════════*FAST FACTS in a NUTSHELL*

Because communication disorders during mild and moderate dementia are complex, nurses should consider a referral for speech therapy to assist in developing a plan to improve communication.

**CLINICAL SNAPSHOT:** Mrs. T has mild dementia and has been admitted for pneumonia. During her hospitalization, you assess that she has significant difficulty with word finding but she tries very hard to communicate and becomes anxious when others do not understand her. When you discuss discharge plans with Mrs. T and her daughter, you suggest that they talk with her doctor about a referral for speech therapy because she has never been evaluated or taught about communication techniques for expressive aphasia.

## Common Issues Occurring During Moderate and Advanced Dementia

Dementia initially affects skills related to language and information processing and gradually affects all aspects of verbal and nonverbal communication. Even in the most advanced stages, however, we need to assume that the person retains some understanding of verbal and nonverbal messages that we communicate. During moderate and advanced dementia, the following communication difficulties occur:

• Repetitious use of phrases, words, or sounds
• Misinterpretation of verbal and nonverbal communication

- Retained ability to talk about familiar experiences of childhood and earlier adulthood, even in the absence of ability to talk about recent events
- Increased difficulty understanding written or verbal communication, progressing to total inability
- Increased difficulty understanding nonverbal communication, but not to the point of total inability
- Reversion to the language used during childhood and younger adulthood or a mix of languages if English is a second language

$=$*FAST FACTS in a NUTSHELL*

Dementia gradually affects all communication abilities, but even during advanced dementia, people are able to perceive messages that are communicated.

⚙ **CLINICAL SNAPSHOT:** Mrs. H, who has advanced dementia, repeatedly cries, "Help me, help me, I need to see her, I need to see her" when she is alone. When she is in a wheelchair near the nurses' station, she is quiet and less anxious because nurses and other staff frequently stop to touch her arm and reassure her that her daughter is coming soon.

## ACTIONS TO IMPROVE VERBAL COMMUNICATION

Nurses routinely adapt their level of communication to the abilities of their patients, but this is very challenging when caring for people with dementia. Nurses can ask families and care partners about helpful communication techniques that have been used prior to hospitalization so these can be incorporated in the care plan. People with mild dementia may be able to tell you what techniques improve their ability to communicate. Some guidelines for communicating with people with dementia are:

- Avoid oversimplification for people with mild dementia but use simpler sentences for people with moderate or advanced dementia.
- Assess the person's response to your communication by observing their verbal and nonverbal responses.
- Document effective and ineffective communication techniques in the care plan.
- Do not talk about a person with dementia as if they were not present.
- Assess the ability of the person with dementia to be included in discussions related to their care and include them appropriately.
- When discussions are about—rather than with—someone with dementia, hold these conversations out of hearing range of the person who is being talked about.
- If the person's hearing is impaired, make sure hearing aids are in place and functional and use effective communication techniques.
- If the person has eyeglasses, make sure they are clean and being used.
- Accept that you may hear the same story repeatedly and this is OK.
- Involve a speech/language therapist for evaluation and management.

Table 12.1 lists examples of specific communication techniques that may be helpful for people with dementia.

## TABLE 12.1  Techniques for Communicating With People With Dementia

| Communication Technique | Example |
| --- | --- |
| Present only one idea at a time. | "We are going shopping now." (Do not add details about stopping for lunch or doing other tasks until the first activity is in process.) |
| Allow time for processing. | Silently count to 10 after asking a question. |
| Use positive statements for directions. | Rather than stating "Don't get out of bed without help," say "Please call for help when you need to get out of bed." |
| Find out if there are certain key words that the person uses in reference to daily activities. | A person with moderate dementia refers to all meals as "lunch" and says "gotta gotta gotta" when she needs to be directed to the bathroom. |
| When discussing activities of daily living, avoid statements that may be interpreted as judgmental. | Rather than stating "You need a bath today," say "It's time for your bath." |
| Rephrase statements that may be interpreted as placing the "blame" on the person with dementia. | Instead of stating "Your words are all so jumbled, you don't make any sense," say "I'm having trouble understanding your words, can you try another word?" |
| Paraphrase or use other words if the person does not understand the first communication. | If the person does not comprehend "Tomorrow you'll be transferred to Sunny View Healthcare Center," say "Tomorrow you're going to another place for more therapy." |
| Assist with word finding and clarify questionable words. | In response to "I don't know what my homework is?" (from a person with moderate dementia after returning from an X-ray), say "Are you wanting to know about the test you just had?" |

*(continued)*

### TABLE 12.1 (continued)

| Communication Technique | Example |
|---|---|
| Do not ask questions that you know the person cannot answer, but give clues to the correct information. | If a patient with moderate dementia has not been able to state the name of the hospital, incorporate that information during usual conversations (e.g., "Is your daughter coming today to see you here at Centerville Hospital?") |
| Make sure all environmental cues provide accurate information. | Keep dry erase boards up to date, make sure clocks and watches are set for correct time. |
| Involve the person in decisions to the best of his or her ability by offering simple and concrete choices. | Say "Do you want chicken or steak?" rather than "What do you want to eat?" |
| Be specific and give one command at a time if the person can follow only one step at a time. | Separate commands, with time between to perform each step: "Pick up this toothbrush … lift it to your mouth … brush your teeth." |
| Do not argue with or correct the person unless it is a matter of safety. | If the person tells you he is going to the ballgame this afternoon, but you know this is not true, do not challenge his statement unless he tries to leave. |
| Try to identify and respond to the person's feelings rather than simply stating facts. | If the person says her mother must be very busy because she has not visited today (and you know her mother is deceased), say "You must be missing her. What is a favorite memory of things you used to do with her?" |
| Ask simple questions to get to know the person behind the dementia. | While you are assisting with patient care, ask "So, what do you do to keep your life interesting?" |
| Use clues in the person's environment to initiate positive communication. | If you see flowers with a card, say something like "These are beautiful flowers from your daughter and her family. They must love you a lot. Do you see them very much?" |

========= *FAST FACTS in a NUTSHELL*

Nurses can assess patient communication patterns and adapt communication techniques to meet the needs of the person with dementia.

💠 **CLINICAL SNAPSHOT:**  The care plan for Mrs. A, who has moderate dementia, incorporates the following interventions, based on the nursing assessment: Provide bedpan when patient says "potty, potty, potty"; ask about two simple choices for liquid nourishment and meal selection; make sure Mrs. A has hearing aid in place when discussing care issues.

## COMMUNICATING RESPECTFULLY

Many people, including nurses, are inclined to "talk down" to people who are cognitively impaired and depend on others to meet their daily needs. This style of communication is easy to slip into when caring for people whose needs are similar to those of infants and children, but it is disrespectful for adults. In addition, we need to pay attention to our tone of voice and inflection and use the same communication style as we would with adults who are cognitively intact. Another communication habit that can be perceived as disrespectful is the inaccurate use of plural pronouns rather than addressing individuals, as in "It's time to take our pills," or "How are we feeling today?" Even terms that are viewed as endearing, such as "honey" or "dearie," are inappropriate when used for adults in care settings. Nurses and all care partners for people with dementia need to self-assess their communication patterns and edit any terms that are associated with infants, children, or loss of control over one's own decisions. Table 12.2 lists examples of these kinds of terms along with appropriate alternatives that can be applied to communication with all older adults.

═══════════════════════════*FAST FACTS in a NUTSHELL*

Nurses communicate respect for people with dementia by avoiding the use of words that are associated with dependency or loss of decision-making abilities.

🔄 **CLINICAL SNAPSHOT:** Mrs. V's son says "I sure dread having to put her in a nursing home." You respond with "It would be a good idea to look at the many places where she could be admitted for the care she requires. There are some very good dementia-care facilities that support the person's dignity and best level of functioning."

---

**TABLE 12.2 Communicating Respectfully With Older Adults**

| Terms to Avoid | Respectful Terms |
| --- | --- |
| Diaper | Brief, incontinence product |
| Bib | Clothing protector |
| Feeding | Dining, eating, meals |
| Caretaker, care giver | Helper, companion, assistant |
| Nursing home | Care facility, rehab center, skilled care center |
| Day care | Day center, day program |
| Nursing home "placement" or "putting in" a nursing home | Admitting for long-term care, or skilled nursing, or rehabilitation |

## NONVERBAL COMMUNICATION

As dementia progresses into moderate and advanced stages, nonverbal communication becomes increasingly important. This holds true for messages being sent both to and from the person with dementia. Thus, an important nursing responsibility is to pay close attention to what you communicate nonverbally—even unintentionally—as well as to what the person with dementia is attempting to communicate. Guidelines for nonverbal communication during moderate and advanced dementia are:

- Assume that all nonverbal expressions of the person with dementia are attempts to communicate needs or feelings.
- Closely observe all nonverbal cues exhibited by the person, especially those that express feelings.
- Assume that even in advanced dementia the person will perceive and understand nonverbal communication, such as touch.
- Be aware of your own nonverbal communication during all interactions, even when the person with dementia is observing you from a distance.
- Assume that your nonverbal cues will communicate more than your spoken words and will be interpreted from the perspective of the person with dementia.

Table 12.3 provides example of nonverbal communication techniques that nurses can use for people with dementia.

### TABLE 12.3 Nonverbal Communication Techniques When Caring for People With Dementia

| Nonverbal Communication Technique | Example |
| --- | --- |
| Attract the person's attention before speaking. | Use direct eye contact, or appropriate touching. |
| Face-to-face positioning at or slightly below eye level. | If the person is sitting or in bed, then sit in a chair opposite the person. |
| Pay attention to your facial expressions. | Use relaxed, smiling expressions; avoid expressions of anxiety or frustration (even if that's what you feel). |

(continued)

**TABLE 12.3 (continued)**

| Nonverbal Communication Technique | Example |
|---|---|
| Reinforce verbal communication with nonverbal communication that is consistent with your message. | When you want someone with moderate dementia to comb his hair, put the comb in his hand and mimic combing your hair. |
| Use simple pictures rather than written words. | Place a picture of a toilet on the bathroom door. |
| Find out how the person responds to touch and use it appropriately. | Use gentle touch to gain the person's attention or reinforce feelings of concern, unless the person responds negatively to being touched. |
| Be aware of possible misinterpretation of your body language. | Avoid facial expressions or arm positions that communicate disapproval such as scowling, wrinkled eyebrows, arms folded across chest, or arms out and on both hips. |

## FAST FACTS in a NUTSHELL

Nurses can use nonverbal communication purposefully when caring for people with dementia.

**CLINICAL SNAPSHOT:** When administering medications to Mr. R, who has moderate dementia, stand face-to-face, establish eye contact, place a cup of water in one of his hands, and ask him to open his other hand. After putting pills in his hand, demonstrate that he is to put the pills into his mouth and then drink the water.

## RESOURCES in a NUTSHELL

*Hartford Institute for Geriatric Nursing*

*consultgerirn.org*

- Communication difficulties: Assessment and interventions in hospitalized older adults with dementia, *Try This*, Issue D7, article and video

# Managing Dementia-Associated Behaviors

# 13

# Dementia-Associated Behaviors

## INTRODUCTION

*The term "dementia-associated behavior" refers to behavioral problems that occur in people with dementia, but this does not mean they are inevitable. Rather, the effects of dementia increase the person's vulnerability to these behaviors, and it is the responsibility of care partners to identify and address the contributing conditions. Because unfamiliar environments or stressful conditions precipitate or exacerbate these behaviors, nurses frequently need to address behavioral issues in their care plans for people with dementia. Examples of behaviors that occur frequently or intermittently during the course of dementia are:*

- *Mrs. M, who has mild dementia, sneaks candy from the shelves when her daughter takes her to the grocery store and is at risk for being caught for shoplifting.*
- *Mr. P lives with his niece and believes she is stealing all his money and using it for her family.*

- Ms. B gets agitated and will not cooperate when she has to change her clothes or take a bath.
- Mr. T strikes out at the nursing assistant when she is assisting him off the commode.
- Mrs. H gets out of bed unassisted and trips over the chair; she rarely remembers to call for help.
- Ms. Q repeatedly calls "Help me, help me, help me, someone please help me" in a distressing tone of voice.

*This chapter focuses on nursing responsibilities pertinent to assessing and addressing behavioral issues when caring for people with dementia. It begins with a discussion of myths and realities, because this is one of the most misunderstood aspects of caring for people with dementia. Content focuses on aspects of care that nurses can address in clinical settings, including tips for teaching family and care partners about dementia-associated behaviors.*

In this chapter, you will learn:

1. Myths and realities related to dementia-associated behaviors
2. Description of behaviors arising from altered perception of reality
3. Causes of dementia-associated behaviors
4. How to assess causes and effects of dementia-associated behaviors
5. Nursing interventions
6. Guidelines for pharmacologic interventions
7. How to address aggressive behaviors

## MYTHS AND REALITIES

An accurate interpretation of dementia-associated behaviors is based on knowledge not only about the person with dementia but also about potential contributing causes. Families, care partners, nurses, and others who care for people with dementia hold many myths and misunderstandings about dementia-associated behaviors. Some myths arise out of generalizations about people with dementia, such as "People with dementia get violent." Misunderstandings also can arise out of personal relationships because it is difficult for spouses and other family members to distinguish between long-term personality patterns and behaviors arising from dementia. This is especially challenging when the person with dementia has a history of dysfunctional behaviors or unhealthy relationships. In these situations, nurses are likely to hear comments such as "He's always manipulated me to get what he wants and now he is better than ever at these tactics." Nurses can help families understand these behaviors by dispelling myths and misunderstandings. In addition, we need to avoid terminology that perpetuates misunderstanding, and accurately assess and address dementia-associated behaviors in our care plans. Table 13.1 summarizes some common misperceptions and related facts about dementia-associated behaviors.

**TABLE 13.1 Misperceptions and Realities About Dementia-Associated Behaviors**

| Misperceptions of Behaviors | Realities |
|---|---|
| "He refuses to ..." | He has no idea about what is offered; needs to do something else before agreeing to the activity; wants to feel he has a choice; may not have ability to carry out the activity. |
| "She fights me when I ..." | She may be experiencing pain or discomfort, which is exacerbated by the activity; she may not understand the activity. |
| Challenging or disruptive behavior | The behavior is a way to cope, adapt, respond, or express a need. |
| "He denies any problem." | He may not have insight, awareness, or ability to understand. |
| "There's no reason for him to act that way." | There usually is a triggering event or an unmet need. |

*(continued)*

**TABLE 13.1  Misperceptions and Realities About Dementia-Associated Behaviors** (*continued*)

| Misperceptions of Behaviors | Realities |
| --- | --- |
| Manipulative, deliberate actions to get attention | Probably does not have enough insight or intent to be manipulative; may be the only way the person is able to express needs. |
| "There's nothing to do to prevent the behavior ..." | Care partners can be proactive in addressing triggers. |
| Thinking that interventions that were effective in the past will continue to be effective | If the usual interventions no longer work, be flexible, creative, and try something else; use a "trial and error" approach by trying variations of interventions that worked. |

## FAST FACTS in a NUTSHELL

Nurses can teach families about the realities of dementia-associated behaviors and avoid terminology or actions that perpetuate myths and misunderstandings (Table 13.1).

## ALTERED PERCEPTION OF REALITY

People with dementia, especially during moderate and later stages, experience altered perceptions of reality in many ways. Health care professionals use the following labels to describe these behaviors:

- *Disoriented to person, place, or time:* cannot give accurate answers when asked to state name of self or familiar people; name of current location or own address; or time of day, month, or season.
- *Delusions:* false beliefs (e.g., "he thinks he's on a boat," "she thinks she has to get to her job," "she took her roommate's shoes because she thought they were hers").
- *Hallucinations:* sensory perceptions not based on actual stimuli (e.g., hearing voices or seeing images not seen by others; tasting or smelling without having corresponding stimuli).

Although these labels originally were applied to manifestations of schizophrenia and other psychiatric conditions, they continue to be used in reference to people with dementia. One consequence of this "labeling system" is that some interventions developed for psychiatric patients are applied to people with dementia. Although dementia experts have questioned the accuracy of these terms for people with dementia, there is no consensus on alternative terms.

The phrase *altered perception of reality* refers to a continuum of symptoms, ranging from relatively simple misperceptions and illusions to more severe delusions and hallucinations. Effects of these misperceptions also vary, ranging from annoyances to severe anxiety and risks to safety.

## Simple Misperceptions of Reality

People with mild dementia experience altered perceptions of reality that are harmless—although annoying and distressing—because of memory deficits, language problems, and other cognitive impairments. Table 13.2 describes misperceptions of reality that are likely to occur in people with dementia.

Simple misperceptions do not necessarily need to be corrected and sometimes the best intervention is to overlook them. Even when misperceptions are harmless, however, nurses need to assess and document these as indicators of mental status. For example, a change in orientation can be an early manifestation of infection or electrolyte imbalance. Nurses need to address misperceptions under the following circumstances:

- They represent a change in mental status that requires further assessment.
- They cause distress or anxiety for the person with dementia or others.
- The person with dementia or others are going to take inappropriate action based on the misperception.
- The misperception poses a risk to the person with dementia or others.

## TABLE 13.2 Misperceptions of Reality That Commonly Occur in People With Dementia

| Misperception | Example |
|---|---|
| Substituted words | "She threw (put) me into bed"; "my mother (daughter) is coming soon." |
| Confabulation: presenting false information as reality | "My daughter is buying a house for me in Florida and I'll be moving there next week" (no basis in reality). |
| Disorientation to person; misperception of family member | "This is my sister" (referring to wife). |
| Disorientation to place | "I live at 224 Saybrook County" (giving incorrect address). |
| Disorientation to time | "It's 1921." |
| Visual illusion: misperception of a visual cue | Thinking the people on television are actually present. |
| Auditory illusion: misperception of an auditory cue | "My daughter is calling for me" (when the person hears nurses talking in the hallway). |

## Delusions

Although delusions are defined as fixed false beliefs, the details may vary from day to day in people with dementia. People with dementia develop delusions primarily because of progressive cognitive impairments and not because of psychosis. Common themes of delusions in people with dementia are:

- People stealing their money or belongings
- Feeling lost or abandoned
- Feeling locked in ("Call the police.")
- Needing to perform a task (taking care of children, going to work)
- Spousal unfaithfulness

These beliefs arise out of the person's distorted perceptions and impaired ability to process and remember information.

Nurses should describe the misperceptions of people with dementia rather than labeling these behaviors as "delusional," "paranoia," or "suspiciousness."

═══════════════════════════════════════ *FAST FACTS in a NUTSHELL*

Delusions may be a way of explaining reality for the person with dementia.

🌀 CLINICAL SNAPSHOT: Mr. C's son has assumed all responsibility for financial management because his father is no longer able to write checks or keep track of his bank accounts. Mr. C tells you that his son has stolen all his money and keeps all his retirement checks.

## Hallucinations

Hallucinations are sensory perceptions that have no basis in reality. Hallucinations can be associated with any of the five senses, but the most common types in people with dementia are visual and auditory, as in the following examples:

• Mrs. M points out the window and says "That person by the tree told me I need to go home right now" (nobody is visible outside).
• Mr. R is alone in his room but states that his son is visiting him.
• Ms. B is petting her cat who sits on her lap (nothing is on her lap).

Visual hallucinations are a prominent feature of Lewy body dementia and they tend to be more vivid than those experienced by people with other types of dementia. Another difference is that hallucinations develop early with Lewy body dementia and later or not at all with Alzheimer's disease.

Hallucinations in people with Lewy body dementia can be exacerbated by conditions such as stress, illness, anesthesia, infections, and physiologic alterations.

# CAUSES OF DEMENTIA-ASSOCIATED BEHAVIORS

Dementia-associated behaviors arise from a combination of factors, including progressive cognitive impairments, environmental conditions, interpersonal factors, and pathologic changes of dementia.

## Progressive Cognitive Impairments

Impaired cognition is the major underlying cause of dementia-associated behaviors because dementia compromises one's ability to do all the following:

- Process information
- Remember information
- Recognize objects, places, people
- Communicate verbally
- Identify and meet one's needs
- Ask for help
- Accept assistance
- Express emotions
- Act in socially appropriate ways
- Cope with stressors
- Understand and manage one's environment

As these cognitive functions decline, usual coping and social skills diminish and the person increasingly relies on nonverbal and behavioral methods to communicate. Thus, many dementia-associated behaviors are attempts to meet physical and emotional needs.

═══════════════*FAST FACTS in a NUTSHELL*

It is reasonable to assume that dementia-related behaviors are expressions of unmet needs due to the person's inability to communicate in other ways.

## Personal Environmental Conditions

Because dementia impairs one's ability to interpret and respond to environmental stimuli, any of the following conditions can significantly affect behaviors in people with dementia:

- Noise: type and sound level of music or television; sirens; sounds from medical equipment; vocalizations from other people with dementia; and voices in the background, even those that are barely audible
- Lighting: glare; lighting that is too dim or too bright
- Familiarity: new place; lack of cues (e.g., photos of self and family); perceived threats (e.g., medical equipment, monitoring devices)
- Temperature: too hot or too cold
- Level of stimulation: visually or audibly over- or understimulating (e.g., monotonous, boring, cluttered, or distracting)
- Colors: poor color contrast; over- or understimulating colors and patterns

## Interpersonal Factors

Caregiver approaches—including those of nurses—are one of the most significant influences on behaviors of people with dementia. For example, when caregivers are stressed or hurried, or when they do not adapt their communication appropriately, people with dementia are likely to react with agitation. In contrast, when caregivers are friendly and re-laxed and use effective communication techniques, people with dementia are less likely to exhibit behavioral changes.

## Pathologic Changes of Dementia

Pathologic changes of dementia significantly increase the risk for manifestations that are called *behavioral and psychological symptoms of dementia (BPSD)*, including:

- Mood disturbances: apathy, depression, euphoria, emotional lability
- Psychotic symptoms: delusions, hallucinations
- Agitation: verbal, vocal, or motor activity not directly due to unmet needs
- Personality changes, disinhibition
- Aberrant motor movements: pacing, wandering, rummaging
- Changes in sleep, eating, appetite

These symptoms are caused by pathologic brain changes of dementia and are perhaps the most challenging to address.

## NURSING ASSESSMENT

Nurses are responsible for assessing causes and effects of be-haviors in people with dementia. Dementia-associated behav-iors have varying effects—both for the person with dementia and all the people with whom they relate—ranging from an-noying and bothersome to risky and seriously unsafe. This is an important aspect of assessment because nurses need to im-mediately address behaviors that are unsafe or arise out of un-met needs. On the other hand, it may be appropriate to ignore, tolerate, or even support behaviors that are due to cognitive impairment but do not affect safety, comfort, or quality of life. In all situations, an accurate assessment of both causes and effects is essential for planning appropriate nursing actions. Nurses can use the following kinds of questions to assess dementia-associated behaviors:

- Is the person expressing a physical need?
- Is the person expressing an emotional need?
- Do the behaviors arise primarily out of confusion, lack of awareness, or misperceptions?
- Do the behaviors pose risks or are they unsafe for the person with dementia?
- Are the behaviors distressing or bothersome for the person with dementia?
- Do the behaviors pose risks for people around the person with dementia (e.g., family, care partners, health care providers, or others in the immediate environment)?
- Are the behaviors annoying or bothersome to other people but not to the person with dementia?

## ═══════════════════════════FAST FACTS in a NUTSHELL

It is important to assess both the causes and the effects of dementia-associated behaviors and plan nursing interventions accordingly.

✪ CLINICAL SNAPSHOT: Nurses know that Mrs. N loudly calls "Sink, sink, I'm sinking" when she needs to void, and they assist her immediately because otherwise she will attempt to get out of bed by herself and she is unsteady. As the nurse is assisting, Mrs. N says, "My mother usually helps me but she's at the store now." The nurse responds, "I'm glad I can be here to help."

## NURSING INTERVENTIONS

Management of dementia-associated behaviors often requires an interdisciplinary team approach, with input from families, care partners, and several health care professionals. An important first step is to ask families and care partners about techniques they use to prevent and manage dementia-associated behaviors. This information is essential for identifying interventions that can be incorporated into care plans for people with dementia. Additional key roles for nurses are addressing contributing conditions, addressing emotional needs, modifying the personal environment, and teaching caregivers.

### Addressing Contributing Conditions

Conditions that cause dementia-associated behaviors and are within the realm of usual nursing care include delirium, depression, medical conditions, adverse medication effects, pain, discomfort, and physical distress from any cause. These conditions are discussed in Chapters 2, 3, and 10. If dementia-associated behaviors occur when the person is receiving assistance with activities of daily living, nurses can apply the techniques discussed in Chapter 14.

### Addressing Emotional Needs

A relatively simple—and universally applicable—nursing intervention for addressing emotional needs is to verbally and nonverbally communicate care, concern, and reassurance during all interactions. Chapter 12 presents information about verbal and nonverbal communication methods that nurses can use. Many other chapters (e.g., Chapters 5 and 6) contain information pertinent to addressing emotional needs of people with dementia.

## Modifying the Personal Environment

Although nurses have limited control over patients' environments, some relatively simple actions they can take when caring for people with dementia include:

- Providing blankets (even warmed ones) when patients are cold
- Adjusting lighting in the room
- Adjusting music and television to appropriate channels
- Promoting a "culture of quiet and calm" in and around patient rooms
- Suggesting that family bring in photos and other reminders of loved ones

═════════════════════════*FAST FACTS in a NUTSHELL*

Nurses can address many causes of dementia-associated behaviors by incorporating simple nursing actions, such as approaching patients in a calm and unhurried manner, in their usual care.

## Addressing Misperceptions of Reality

When altered perceptions of reality represent a change in mental status, the first nursing responsibility is to identify conditions that are contributing to the change, as discussed in Chapters 2, 3, and 10. Nurses address altered perceptions through communication methods discussed in Chapter 12. Distraction, or redirection of attention, is often an effective intervention, especially when you can get the person to focus on pleasant, comforting, or health-promoting activities (e.g., music, food, walking, or conversing about happy memories). As with other aspects of caring for people with dementia, nurses can ask families and other care partners about activities that they use for redirecting the person's attention.

Although reorienting people to reality can be therapeutic and helpful, sometimes it is more therapeutic to avoid providing information that can increase the person's distress. For example, people with dementia may forget that a spouse or parent is deceased and they may repeatedly inquire about that person. The traditional reality orientation approach would be to remind them the person is dead, but this is not necessarily appropriate for people with dementia. In these situations, reminders that the person is dead often precipitate new or renewed feelings of grief and many questions about why the person with dementia was not told before. In addition, reorientation may reinforce the person's limitations and add to their distress. Nursing actions to address these kinds of situations include the following:

- Avoid discussion of details but address feelings ("You must miss your mother a lot. Are you feeling sad right now?")
- Distract with questions or activities ("I'm sorry your husband can't be here now. Tell me about your wedding.")
- Communicate a sense of safety ("Your mother isn't here, but she is fine.")
- If the person starts to cry and express sadness or grief, offer support but do not discourage expression of feelings unless the emotions are too distressful or prolonged.
- Use nonverbal communication to promote a sense of calm and caring.

## ═══════════════════════════════════*FAST FACTS in a NUTSHELL*

Identifying the most therapeutic response to address misperceptions of reality is often a "trial and error" process. Nurses can ask families and care partners about interventions that have worked for them and incorporate these into the care plan.

## Teaching Caregivers

When family members or care partners express concern or ask questions about ways they can address behavioral issues, nurses can help them identify and address precipitating conditions. Nurses also can teach about communication techniques, environmental modifications, and other pertinent interventions discussed in this chapter. In addition, nurses can encourage families to consider the following types of interventions that are effective for addressing behaviors and improving the quality of life for people with dementia:

• Hand massage
• Touch therapy
• Music therapy
• Pet therapy
• Physical exercise

Families and care partners can find information about ways of addressing dementia-associated behaviors from the Alzheimer's Association and Internet sites listed in the Resources in a Nutshell section at the end of this chapter.

## AGGRESSIVE BEHAVIORS

People with dementia may exhibit aggressive behaviors such as hitting, biting, slapping, scratching, punching, grabbing, and kicking. Aggressive behaviors are acts that cause harm to or threaten the safety of others, the person with dementia, or objects in the person's environment. Nurses are most likely to encounter these behaviors when they are in close proximity to people with dementia during care activities. Aggressive behaviors usually arise out of confusion as an act to protect oneself from perceived harm or threat. Aggressive behaviors also arise because people with dementia feel little or no control over actions being imposed on them by others.

Nursing interventions focus on preventing aggressive behaviors, protecting all people involved, and de-escalating the behaviors. To achieve these goals nurses can incorporate the following actions in their care plans:

- Ask family members and other care partners about activities that are likely to precipitate aggressive behaviors.
- Identify care-related activities that have caused the person to react aggressively or with significant resistance in the past.
- Incorporate information in care plans about effective ways of preventing aggressive behaviors.
- Avoid conditions that increase anxiety: noise, overstimulating environment, more than one staff approaching or talking with the person.
- Recognize that the person with dementia may be reacting aggressively to a particular staff person, and try to avoid interactions with that staff person.
- Observe for indicators of behaviors escalating toward aggression: muscle tension, raising arms, facial expressions, and vocalizations.
- Step out of the reach of the person with dementia as soon as you observe indicators of potential aggressive acts.
- Use a calm and reassuring voice and demeanor.
- Avoid loud or authoritative tone of voice, but communicate a sense of calm and direction.
- If you feel anxious or are hurried, take time to become centered and calm before and during interactions and patient care activities.
- Clearly and simply describe each step related to care activities before and during your nursing actions.
- When aggression is a reaction to the person's loss of control over his or her care, incorporate interventions that address autonomy and perceived control

(e.g., facilitating as much independence as possible, even when it is more time consuming; asking "Is it OK if I ....").

- Use gentle touch, while also providing appropriate personal space.
- Use nonthreatening actions for self-protection: Use your free hand to pry fingers away when someone grabs your arm.
- Protect yourself by keeping at arms, length or out of reach as much as possible.
- Tell the person that the behavior is unacceptable by using a simple statement ("That hurts, stop kicking").
- Address the feelings of the person with dementia ("This may seem frightening to you, but you are safe and we are helping you to be comfortable in bed").
- When absolutely necessary, use a method of holding the patient to prevent harm; move the person into a safe position as soon as possible.
- Once the person with dementia is in a safe position, have only one staff interact if this is safe for all involved.
- Keep the person's close environment clear of objects that can be thrown, broken, or cause harm.
- Arrange for an interdisciplinary team assessment to develop approaches that may include the use of medications.

When precipitating conditions cannot be identified, or when aggressive behaviors occur frequently and do not seem to be related to care activities, health care professionals need to look for other causes. For example, because aggressive behaviors can be a symptom of delirium, nurses need to consider all causative conditions discussed in Chapter 2. Even in the absence of delirium, conditions that increase the risk for aggressive behaviors in people with dementia include depression, hallucinations, and constipation (Power, 2011). Aggressive behaviors also may be caused by pain or discomfort, even when the person does not appear to be in pain, as discussed in Chapter 10.

================ *FAST FACTS in a NUTSHELL*

When people with dementia exhibit aggressive behaviors, nurses need to address the cause and provide for safety of the person with dementia and others who are involved.

## PHARMACOLOGIC INTERVENTIONS

Although antipsychotics and antianxiety agents have been used for decades for dementia-associated behaviors, there is growing recognition that these medications are not effective and, in fact, can be quite detrimental. Dr. Allen Power summarizes reasons for not using antipsychotics in his book *Dementia Beyond Drugs* (2010):

- For most people with dementia, the risks of antipsychotics outweigh the benefits.
- Reviews of antipsychotic medications consistently conclude that these drugs have very limited effectiveness.
- Effectiveness of antipsychotic medications is due primarily to their sedative qualities, which usually cause increased somnolence and confusion.
- Antipsychotic drugs have been associated with increased mortality in people with dementia.
- All antipsychotic drugs produce sedation, which can cause additional negative consequences.
- Studies of antipsychotic drugs show a very high rate of response to placebos (i.e., there is little difference between treatment and control groups).
- Studies indicate that 30% to 60% of people with behavioral symptoms improve without medications.

Dementia experts consistently have expressed concerns about the low effectiveness and high risk of adverse effects of antipsychotic medications. One review of risk versus benefit concluded that for every 1,000 people with dementia treated with antipsychotics, no more than 20% would improve, but the direct adverse effects would include 10 deaths, 18 vascular events (with half of those being severe), and 60–94 patients with gait disturbances (Banerjee, 2009). Numerous studies have confirmed that antipsychotic medications significantly increase the risk of death, stroke, and transient ischemic events in older adults and people with dementia. All categories of psychotropic medications are associated with an increased risk of death and other serious consequences, but the risk is less for newer (atypical) antipsychotics compared to older (typical) antipsychotics, benzodiazepines, and antidepressants (Huybrechts, Rothman, Siliman, Brookhart, & Schneeweiss, 2011).

## Typical Antipsychotics

Medications developed during the 1970s for treatment of psychosis are referred to as *typical* or first-generation antipsychotics. Haloperidol (Haldol) is the one that has been most commonly used for neuropsychiatric manifestations of dementia. In more recent years, these drugs are rarely used for dementia due to serious adverse effects, which are similar to and more severe than those listed for atypical antipsychotics.

## Atypical Antipsychotics

The most commonly used *atypical* (or second-generation) antipsychotics for dementia-associated behaviors are aripiprazole (Abilify), clozapine (Clozaril), olanzapine (Zyprexa), quetiapine (Seroquel), risperidone (Risperdal), and ziprasidone (Geodon). Adverse effects of atypical antipsychotics include falls, confusion, drowsiness, anticholinergic effects, and increased mortality due to cardiovascular and cerebrovascular events. Short-term use may be necessary and effective for controlling aggression, agitation, and psychotic symptoms, but these medications should be used in the lowest effective dose. A recent review of studies found small but statistically significant improvement in dementia-associated behaviors for aripiprazole, olanzapine, and risperidone (Maher et al., 2011). People with Lewy body dementia are particularly susceptible to effects of psychotropic medications, so the dose should be as low as possible with the longest possible interval between doses.

## Benzodiazepines

The following benzodiazepines are sometimes used to promote sleep and reduce anxiety and agitation in people with dementia: alprazolam (Xanax), lorazepam (Ativan), and clonazepam (Klonipin). Adverse effects that are common and serious in older adults include falls, sedation, increased confusion, tolerance, dependence, and rebound insomnia. Adverse effects are more likely to occur when benzodiazepines are used regularly or long term, or when the medication has a long half-life (e.g., flurazepam [Dalmane]).

## Guidelines for Nurses

Nurses should consider all the following principles related to antipsychotics and benzodiazepines for dementia-associated behaviors:

- Psychotropic medications are a last resort for dementia-associated behaviors and should be initiated only after other measures have been tried and when the behaviors are unsafe or cause serious distress.

- Short-term (up to 12 weeks) use of antipsychotics may be effective for management of severe physical aggression.
- Use lowest effective dose and monitor for adverse effects.
- Adverse effects of antipsychotics include restlessness, incontinence, stroke, dry mouth, constipation, cognitive decline, parkinsonism, diabetes, and depression.
- Review all psychotropic medications at least once every 3 months and consider dose reduction or discontinuation.
- Review all psychotropic medications whenever there is a change in the person's condition or environment (e.g., when admitted to the hospital and upon discharge).
- Health care providers need to carefully weigh the risks versus benefits before initiating pharmacologic interventions.

## Antidepressants

There is much evidence to support the use of antidepressants for people with both dementia and depression; however, these drugs are also associated with significant risks. Selective serotonin reuptake inhibitors (SSRIs) are the type of antidepressant most commonly used for people with dementia. Examples of SSRIs are: citalopram (Celexa), escitalopram (Lexapro), fluvoxamine (Luvox), paroxetine (Paxil), and sertraline (Zoloft). These medications are appropriate for treatment of depression in people with dementia, but they are less effective for dementia-associated behaviors that are not directly caused by depression. One study found that citalopram was effective for agitation and emotional lability, but evidence for overall effectiveness for dementia-associated behaviors is lacking. Nurses should consider all the following principles related to antidepressants for people with dementia:

- Antidepressants are appropriate, and often underutilized, for treatment of depression in people with dementia.

- Antidepressants may alleviate behaviors to the extent that they are due to depression, such as apathy, agitation, irritability, emotional lability, decreased concentration, sleep disturbances, and diminished appetite.
- Immediate improvement will not be evident but the medication should be given a fair trial (i.e., as long as 12 weeks) as long as serious adverse effects do not occur.
- Common adverse effects of antidepressants include nausea, vomiting, diarrhea, headache, nervousness, insomnia, tremor, dry mouth, and sexual dysfunction.
- Antidepressants cannot be used on an "as needed" (prn) basis.

═══════════════════*FAST FACTS in a NUTSHELL*

Pharmacologic interventions are used only as a last resort for dementia-associated behaviors because of their limited efficacy and high risk for adverse effects. When they are prescribed, they should be the lowest dose for the shortest time and nurses need to observe for adverse effects.

═══════════════════*RESOURCES in a NUTSHELL*

*Alzheimer's Association*

*www.alz.org*
- Information for professionals and families about dementia-associated behaviors

*Hartford Institute for Geriatric Nursing*

*consultgerirn.org*
- Therapeutic Activity Kits, *Try This,* Issue D4

# 14

# Issues Related to Daily Activities

## INTRODUCTION

*People with dementia experience problems with performing daily care activities, and they depend on others to assist with their care. People with mild and moderate dementia usually have a routine that enables them to maintain some independence. They often are dependent on a step-by-step process or the provision of cues and verbal prompts. Any change in their environment or caregiver situation can disrupt their routines and increase their dependency on others. Nurses need to identify ways to support the person's ability to perform daily activities as much as possible, even when this is more time consuming than doing the activities for the person.*

In this chapter, you will learn:

1. How to identify the level of assistance that is most appropriate for the person with dementia
2. Nursing interventions to address issues related to eating
3. Nursing interventions to address issues related to bathing, dressing, and personal care

4. How to promote bladder and bowel continence
5. Nursing interventions to facilitate administration of medications and treatments
6. Nursing interventions to promote sleep

## PROVIDING THE APPROPRIATE LEVEL OF CARE

An essential aspect of person-centered care is identifying the level of assistance that is most appropriate for the person with dementia. Nurses routinely assess patients for pain, limitations, response to illness, and all aspects of care that affect their health and functioning. When we care for people with dementia, we need to add another layer of assessment to identify strengths and abilities so we can implement interventions that support the person's highest level of function. Although this may take more time than providing care directly, it is an essential aspect of person-centered care. This approach is also essential for preventing *excess disability*, which refers to limitations that unnecessarily interfere with someone's level of functioning. People with dementia frequently experience excess disability because the people with whom they interact do not understand how to promote their highest level of functioning.

═══════════════════════════*FAST FACTS in a NUTSHELL*

Nurses provide person-centered care and prevent excess disability when they develop a care plan based on an assessment of the person's strengths and abilities.

## ASSESSING COGNITIVE ABILITIES

One's ability to perform daily activities is affected by physical and cognitive skills. Whereas physical skills may be easy to assess, it is more challenging to assess cognitive skills that affect performance of daily activities. Whenever feasible, nurses can facilitate a referral for an occupational therapist to assess abilities and develop care plans for people with dementia. Nurses also can ask families and care partners about interventions that facilitate the person's performance of activities of daily living (ADL). People with mild dementia may be able to describe actions that support their ability to perform ADL as independently as possible. In addition, nurses have many opportunities to assess the person's ability to do the following:

- Initiate a task
- Understand directions
- Perform steps in the correct order
- Maintain attention
- Complete an activity
- Imitate actions of others

Nurses use information about these cognitive skills as a guide to developing care plans that support the optimal level of independence for people with dementia. Nurses can use the communication techniques discussed in Chapter 12 to address cognitive skills that affect performance of daily activities. The next sections of this chapter provide guidelines for addressing the daily activities that are most pertinent to care of people with dementia. Interventions for safe mobility are discussed in Chapter 11.

## ═══════════════════════*FAST FACTS in a NUTSHELL*

Nurses assess cognitive skills and plan interventions that support the person's optimal level of functioning in daily activities. Whenever feasible, nurses can facilitate a referral for an occupational therapist to assess and develop a care plan for people with dementia.

## EATING

Problems with eating occur during all stages of dementia, as illustrated in the following examples:

- Forgetting to eat, beginning during early stages
- Loss of appetite (sometimes due to depression)
- Inability to prepare foods and lack of appropriate assistance or prompts
- Loss of ability to recognize food as something pleasurable
- Not understanding the tasks involved (e.g., not taking lids off containers or not opening individual condiment packages)
- Being in an unfamiliar and confusing environment
- Inability to maintain attention
- Difficulty chewing due to dental problems or not having comfortable dentures
- Difficulty chewing and swallowing due to advanced dementia or other pathologic conditions
- Increased risk of aspiration due to difficulty chewing and swallowing

Managing eating behaviors is an essential aspect of providing adequate nutrition and hydration. These issues are especially complex in the advanced stage of dementia because they involve decisions related to the use of tube feedings, as discussed in Chapter 8.

It is helpful to ask families and care partners about interventions they find effective to promote nutrition for the person with dementia. Particularly effective strategies may include providing favorite foods and serving at the preferred texture or temperature. Nurses also can initiate referrals for dieticians or speech therapists for assessment and interventions related to nutritional needs (including significant weight loss) and techniques for addressing chewing and swallowing difficulties. If patients have difficulty filling out menus or following the procedure for ordering food and beverages, nurses can provide or arrange for appropriate assistance.

Nursing interventions that may be appropriate for addressing eating problems in people with dementia include:

- Opening containers, removing lids, and setting up trays so food items are easily accessible
- Describing food items that the person may not recognize
- Providing small frequent meals
- Offering nutritious snacks and beverages
- Cutting food into bite-size pieces before presenting it
- Sitting face-to-face and using a friendly approach when feeding
- Providing appropriate verbal and nonverbal cues
- Using cups rather than bowls for soups and thin cereals
- Adapting the environment as much as possible to control noise, distractions, and overstimulation

═══════════════*FAST FACTS in a NUTSHELL*

Nurses work closely with families, care partners, dieticians, and speech therapists to identify interventions that are most effective for addressing nutritional needs of people with dementia.

## BATHING, DRESSING, AND PERSONAL CARE

People with dementia are likely to have a routine directed by their care partners that enables them to get dressed and carry out personal care activities in their usual setting. When they do not have their usual cues and routines, they are likely to be confused and less able to perform their daily activities. When nurses and other unfamiliar people assist with their care, they are likely to be resistive or even combative. In addition, people with dementia have difficulty initiating activities and they may be confused about the use of unfamiliar products, such as sealed bath bags. The following nursing interventions may be appropriate when providing personal care for people with dementia:

- Find out what the person's usual routine is and adhere to it as closely as possible (e.g., same time of day, preferred method, best approach).
- Keep the care as simple as possible.
- Assess for pain or discomfort as possible causes of resistance.
- Encourage family or care partners to provide assistance as they usually do.
- Provide for privacy and comfort (e.g., keep the person covered, close bed curtains, and make sure the environment is warm).
- Observe whether the person performs oral care and provide assistance or prompts as necessary.
- Describe your actions in simple terms if the person feels threatened or does not understand what you are doing.
- If the person is physically aggressive or resistive, stop the task and address the behaviors; resume the task only when the person is calm and cooperative.
- Provide prompts for, or appropriate assistance with, hair care and shaving.
- If resources are available, ask care partners if they want to arrange for barber or beautician services.

## ══════════════════════════════ FAST FACTS in a NUTSHELL

People with mild and moderate dementia usually have a routine that enables them to perform personal care activities with prompts, setups, or minimal assistance.

⚙ **CLINICAL SNAPSHOT:** The care plan for Mr. C includes the following intervention: After breakfast and before bed, supervise Mr. C's oral care by putting toothpaste on his toothbrush, placing it on the sink near a cup of water, and verbally prompting him to brush his teeth.

## BOWEL AND BLADDER CONTINENCE

Nursing interventions to help maintain continence can be very challenging because people with dementia gradually lose control of bowel and bladder elimination. Nurses need to assess the person's usual pattern of bowel and bladder elimination and identify conditions that are likely to cause incontinence, such as the following:

- Unfamiliar environments, difficulty finding toileting facilities
- Not receiving timely and appropriate assistance with toileting needs
- Urinary tract infection
- Constipation
- Adverse medication effects (e.g., diuretics, narcotics, anticholinergics)
- Incontinence briefs that interfere with the person's ability to use a commode
- Functional limitations that affect the person's ability to get to a toilet in a timely manner

Even if dementia does not affect one's control over bowel and bladder elimination, it can affect one's ability to remember to use the toilet. Dementia also affects one's ability to report about bowel movements. Nurses can use any of the following strategies to promote continence in people with dementia:

- Observe patterns of bowel and bladder elimination; do not rely on the person to accurately self-report.
- Observe for and respond to signs that the person needs assistance with toileting.
- Develop a care plan for anticipating and addressing toileting needs (usually at 2-hour intervals during the day).
- Document frequency, amount, and consistency of bowel movements and be on the alert for signs of constipation.

- Provide cues and assistance at appropriate intervals.
- Make sure the bathroom is clearly marked and the pathway to it is uncluttered.
- Arrange for medical evaluation for conditions that may contribute to incontinence (e.g., urinary tract infection, enlarged prostate, urinary retention).
- If incontinence occurs, preserve the person's dignity and avoid any responses that may seem judgmental or patronizing.
- Provide assistance with or reminders about hand washing after using the bathroom.

## ═══════════════════════════════════════ FAST FACTS in a NUTSHELL

It is important to identify factors that affect bowel and bladder continence for each patient with dementia and plan individualized interventions to prevent episodes of incontinence.

**CLINICAL SNAPSHOT:** Mrs. G's care plan includes the following: Patient becomes agitated if incontinence briefs are used; provide verbal prompts and stand-by assistance with walking to the bathroom every 3 hours during the day and once during the night when she is awake; observe toilet for stool and record in chart.

## MEDICATIONS AND TREATMENTS

When nurses administer medications, take vital signs, or perform other direct care activities for patients who have dementia, they often deal with challenges such as:

- Refusal to take medications because the person believes they are poison, or for other reasons not based in reality
- Difficulty swallowing medications

- Diminished ability or inability to understand directions or explanations
- Fear or perception of threat in relation to invasive procedures (i.e., blood draws, injections)
- Fear of or experience of pain or discomfort due to being moved or repositioned
- Misperceptions of medical equipment

When people with dementia are resistant, or even combative, nurses need to address conditions that contribute to fear and misperceptions, as discussed in Chapter 13. Additional interventions to facilitate direct care include the following:

- Ask families and care partners about effective approaches that they use.
- Offer medications with a simple statement, such as "It's time for you to have these." Use verbal and nonverbal prompts as appropriate.
- Unless contraindicated (e.g., enteric coated or extended release), crush medications and put in small amount of soft food that the person likes.
- If the person resists or has difficulty swallowing pills, consult with pharmacist about forms of medications that are most acceptable (e.g., liquid, dissolving tablets, or patches).
- Do not argue with the person, but use a direct and reassuring approach.
- Address pain and comfort conditions that may be causing resistance or refusal.
- If the person pulls at tubes, cover the tubing with loose fluffy bandages.
- Obtain assistance from family or staff to distract the person's attention while you are checking vital signs or performing nursing procedures.
- If the person is resistive or agitated, perform the care task at another time.
- If feasible, perform nursing procedures at the time of day when the person is usually more cooperative.

**==FAST FACTS in a NUTSHELL**

Creative strategies are often needed for administering medications and treatments to people with dementia.

⭐ **CLINICAL SNAPSHOT:** Mrs. G's daughter reports that her mother takes her pills if you crush them, put them in vanilla pudding, provide a cup of warm water, and say, "This is the pudding that Molly made for you and it has your pills in it to make you feel better."

## SLEEP

At least half of people with dementia experience significant sleep disturbances, such as

- Day–night sleep pattern reversal
- Frequent nighttime awakenings
- Fragmented sleep patterns
- Excessive daytime sleepiness
- Increased somnolence (15 or more hours/day, especially in very advanced dementia)

People with Lewy body dementia are especially apt to develop sleep disturbances, and these may occur even before the onset of cognitive changes. The two most prominent sleep disorders in people with Lewy body dementia are (1) very active dreaming (i.e., very active body movements, even becoming violent, during dreams) and (2) excessive daytime sleepiness.

Sleep disturbances are caused by dementia-associated brain changes and concomitant conditions including pain, anxiety, delirium, depression, sleep apnea, medical conditions, restless legs syndrome, and adverse medication effects.

As with all conditions in people with dementia, nurses need to identify factors that contribute to sleep disturbances rather than attribute the problem solely to dementia. For example, nurses can assess and address pain in people with dementia, as discussed in Chapter 10. Nurses also can talk with primary care practitioners to address medical conditions or adverse medication effects that can cause sleep disturbances.

LaReau, Benson, Watcharotone, and Manguba (2008) identified the following relatively simple nursing actions that improved sleep in hospitalized older adults, which are listed in order of patient preferences:

- Assisting with personal hygiene (e.g., toileting, mouth care)
- Adhering to usual bedtime
- Providing a 5-minute head-to-toe massage
- Straightening bed linens
- Providing a bedtime snack
- Minimizing bedside conversation
- Darkening the room

Another intervention that may be effective for people with dementia is asking someone to stay with the person to provide comfort and reassurance.

If pharmacologic interventions are necessary for sleep disturbances, nurses need to be aware of the increased risk of serious adverse effects in older adults with dementia, as discussed in Chapter 13. Nonbenzodiazepine hypnotics that are recommended for short-term use for insomnia are: eszopiclone (Lunesta), ramelteon (Rozerem), zaleplon (Sonata), and zolpidem (Ambien). Nurses caring for people with sleep disorders due to Lewy body dementia should discuss this problem with their neurologist because of the unique characteristics of this type of dementia (including their atypical reactions to medications).

Nurses can teach nonpharmacologic interventions that promote sleep such as the following:

- Try to maintain a regular daily schedule for sleep, rest, activity, and meals.
- Take a warm, relaxing bath in the afternoon or early evening.
- Encourage regular daily exercise and interesting physical activities.
- Address pain, anxiety, distress, and any other sources of discomfort.
- Encourage exposure to sunlight or full-spectrum lighting during the day.
- After 1 p.m., avoid foods, beverages, and medications that contain caffeine or stimulants (e.g., tea, cocoa, coffee, chocolate, sugar, refined carbohydrates, and some over-the-counter pain relievers and cold preparations).
- In the evening drink beverages and eat snacks that promote sleep (e.g., warm milk, chamomile tea, and snacks with whole grains).
- Listen to soothing music.
- Make sure bedroom temperature is comfortable.
- Control lighting and noise for optimal sleep conditions.
- In the evening and if the person wakens during the night, avoid activities that are stimulating or confusing (e.g., television, distracting conversations).
- Use lavender essential oil for aromatherapy.
- Use one or more of the following relaxation methods: imagery, meditation, deep breathing, progressive relaxation, body or foot massage, or rocking in a chair.

================*FAST FACTS in a NUTSHELL*

Developing and incorporating relatively simple interventions known to be effective from family or caregivers
can be useful in promoting sleep.

**⚙ CLINICAL SNAPSHOT:** When Mr. N's son visits him in
the evening, nurses bring chamomile tea from the bever-
age cart so the son can encourage him to drink it.

================*RESOURCES in a NUTSHELL*

*Bathing Without a Battle: Person-Directed Care of
Individuals With Dementia* by A. L. Barrick, J. Rader,
B. Hoeffer, P. D. Sloane, & S. Biddle (Eds.), New York, NY:
Springer Publishing Company, 2008.

# Broader Aspects of Care for People With Dementia

# 15

## Ethical and Legal Issues

### INTRODUCTION

*Supporting the rights of the person with dementia is one of the greatest challenges—and a core aspect—of person-centered care. During the course of dementia, many questions arise about the person's rights to carry out activities that become risky or unsafe because of cognitive impairments. These issues typically arise during mild and moderate dementia and continue until people with dementia are no longer able to participate in decisions about their care. During advanced dementia, additional issues arise related to decisions about medical interventions and goals of care, as discussed in Chapter 8. Nurses can address these issues by considering ethical and legal guidelines as discussed in this chapter.*

In this chapter, you will learn:

1. Nursing considerations related to decisional capacity in people with dementia
2. Nursing responsibilities related to legal documents for people with dementia
3. How to address elder abuse and neglect

## RIGHTS OF PEOPLE WITH DEMENTIA

People do not lose any rights solely because they have dementia, but when their decision-making abilities are significantly impaired, they increasingly rely on others to protect them from harm. In the ideal situation, the person has all legal documents in order and has supportive family and care partners who make decisions that are acceptable to the person with dementia. However, ethical issues often arise because of lack of appropriate legal documents, disagreements among surrogate decision makers, or resistance on the part of the person with dementia. In these situations, nurses and other health care providers are likely to be involved with decisions involving freedom versus safety for the person with dementia. Sometimes the decisions relate to a situation that is not harmful in itself but poses a risk for harm. These situations involve weighing the person's freedom and safety against probable or possible harm. Many of these issues are associated with daily activities and loss of roles and responsibilities that the person carried out independently for many years, as illustrated by the following examples:

- Driving a vehicle
- Living alone
- Refusing or resisting assistance with activities of daily living
- Cooking independently, even when the person frequently burns food
- Managing medications independently, even when it is not done reliably
- Refusing or resisting a move to a safer environment
- Refusing or resisting medical care
- Managing finances independently
- Walking independently, even with unsafe mobility
- Going outside one's home, even when the person is likely to get lost
- Smoking independently, even with the risk of fires

These issues are addressed, in part, by assessing the decisional capacity of the person with dementia, which is usually done by several health care professionals, including nurses. In addition, nurses can facilitate referrals for the following health care professionals:

- Occupational therapist: assessment and rehabilitation services related to driving and other activities that may be risky
- Physical therapist: assessment and therapy for balance and mobility
- Speech therapist: assessment and interventions related to memory, cognition, and communication
- Psychologist or social worker: assessment and interventions to address resistance, conflicts, and coping
- Social worker or geriatric care manager: referrals for legal and financial professionals who specialize in eldercare issues

═══════════════════════════*FAST FACTS in a NUTSHELL*

Nurses address decisions about issues related to daily activities by suggesting referrals for appropriate health care professionals and facilitating communication among all team members.

## ASSESSING DECISIONAL CAPACITY

All competent adults have the right to direct their own lives as long as their actions do not infringe on the rights of others, but they can lose this right if they do not have *decisional capacity*. People who have decisional capacity must be able to do all the following:

- Understand relevant information
- Demonstrate comprehension of the information
- Apply the information to one's own situation

- Consider alternatives and the associated consequences
- Communicate the decision to others
- Take appropriate actions to implement the decision

Decisional capacity is usually determined in relation to a particular situation and it differs from *competency*, which is a legal term that refers to the ability to fulfill one's roles and handle one's affairs in a responsible manner.

Nurses are involved with assessment of decisional capacity when signatures are required for procedures and at many other times when they care for people with dementia. The following are important points to consider when discussing decisions about care:

- People with mild and moderate dementia usually retain some decision-making capacity.
- Make arrangements if the person would like to involve other people in the discussion.
- Adapt your communication to the person's abilities, as discussed in Chapter 12.
- Present the information in the most understandable terms.
- Allow time for the person to consider the information.
- Encourage the person to ask questions.
- Obtain feedback to assess the person's understanding.
- Discuss the information ahead of time with trusted family members or surrogate decision makers and plan the best way to involve the person with dementia.
- Address conditions that can interfere with communication (e.g., ensuring that a hearing-impaired person uses his or her hearing aid).
- Plan discussions as much as possible when the person is rested, alert, and comfortable.
- When you have questions about the person's ability, ask another nurse to reassess at another time.
- If appropriate, involve other health care professionals.

Nurses have key roles in assessing decisional capacity, but it is important to request evaluations from other health care professionals when the situation is unclear or when conflicts arise. This is especially important when major decisions are being made that affect the person's right to self-determination.

═══════════════════════*FAST FACTS in a NUTSHELL*

Nurses have key roles in assessing decisional capacity and in facilitating referrals for other health care professionals (e.g., geriatricians, psychologists, psychiatrists, and social workers).

## ESSENTIAL LEGAL DOCUMENTS

One of the most important aspects of caring for people with dementia is ensuring that legal documents are in place before issues arise about competency or decisional capacity. The Alzheimer's Association and dementia experts emphasize the importance of executing these legal documents as soon as the diagnosis has been made. Even when cognitive abilities are compromised, people with dementia may be capable of executing legal documents as long as they are able to understand the issues and communicate their intentions. Legal documents most pertinent to health care situations are the durable power of attorney for health care, living wills, and medical directives.

### Durable Power of Attorney for Health Care

A durable power of attorney for health care is a legally binding document that takes effect whenever someone—for any reason—cannot provide informed consent for health care treatment decisions. Because this document authorizes a surrogate decision maker (also called a health care proxy) to represent the person during any time of incapacity, it is often considered the most important legal document. A durable power of attorney for health care must be initiated when the person is competent, and it takes effect only when the person is incapacitated. Nurses are responsible for documenting information about the person's legally appointed surrogate decision makers and for including them in discussions and decisions about care.

The primary responsibility of the surrogate decision maker is to make and support decisions that are consistent with the wishes of the person with dementia. Ideally, these wishes have been documented in advance directives, and it is imperative that the health care proxy have a copy of all advance directives and periodically discuss the person's wishes. Even when the wishes are documented, these decisions are not always clear, and the surrogate decision maker may experience emotional turmoil about the decisions. Nurses often assume advisory roles in clarifying information and supporting the health care power of attorney when decisions are difficult.

## ═══════════════════════════════════════ *FAST FACTS in a NUTSHELL*

Nurses provide information and support for surrogate decision makers.

✪ **CLINICAL SNAPSHOT:** Mrs. H's cardiologist has scheduled surgery for a pacemaker and you are responsible for obtaining informed consent. Mrs. H has advanced dementia and her daughter, who is her surrogate decision maker, tells you she isn't sure if her mother would want to have this done because she always said "When it's my time, God will take me and I don't want any doctors or anyone else interfering with that plan." You give the daughter written information about the risks and benefits of the procedure and you arrange for her to discuss this with the doctor.

If this legal document has not been executed, spouses, adult children, and other close relatives often assume decision-making responsibilities for the person with dementia. When conflicts arise among those who assume decision-making responsibilities and the person with dementia is not capable of making these decisions, more restrictive legal actions, such as guardianship, may be necessary. When nurses are aware of conflicts about decisions, they need to document this information and discuss this with other members of the health care team.

## Living Wills

Living wills are advance directives that allow people to specify the type of medical treatment they would want or not want if they become incapacitated as a result of terminal illness. These documents affirm the right of a person to refuse treatment, but they do not always specify the particular type of treatment that can be refused. In addition, they can document the person's preferences about pain management, organ donation, place of death, and specific treatments he or she would want to receive. Living wills apply only when the person is terminally ill, and this may be difficult to determine, particularly during advanced dementia (as discussed in Chapter 8).

## Medical Directives

A do-not-resuscitate (DNR) order is a very specific type of advance directive that compels health care providers to refrain from cardiopulmonary resuscitation if the person is no longer breathing and has no heartbeat. Some states allow variations of the DNR order, with the most common one being Comfort Care DNR (also called DNR-Comfort Care, CC/DNR, or Comfort Care Only DNR). These legal documents direct health care professionals to provide designated comfort care measures but not resuscitative therapies. In addition to addressing DNR interventions, medical directives can address specific interventions, such as antibiotics, food and nutrition, and admission to the hospital. These documents should be reviewed periodically, especially during advanced dementia, as discussed in Chapter 8.

## ════════════════════════════════*FAST FACTS in a NUTSHELL*

Nurses initiate discussions of advance directives when they care for people with dementia, document these discussions, and ensure that all pertinent documents are available for all health care professionals.

## ELDER ABUSE AND NEGLECT

Dementia increases the risk for self-neglect and elder abuse and neglect, so nurses need to be alert to this possibility and take appropriate actions. Elder abuse occurs under any of the following circumstances:

- A caregiver or other responsible person performs acts that cause or create a serious risk of harm to a vulnerable older adult (e.g., physical abuse, sexual abuse, emotional or psychological abuse, and financial or material exploitation).
- A caregiver or other responsible person fails to satisfy the elder's basic needs or to protect the elder from harm (e.g., neglect, abandonment).
- The behaviors of older adults threaten their health or safety (self-neglect).

Impaired judgment, lack of insight, inability to make safe decisions, and misperceptions of reality are dementia-associated characteristics that can lead to abuse and neglect. One study found that 47.3% of a sample of 129 persons with dementia were mistreated by their caregivers (Wiglesworth et al., 2010). Variables associated with increased occurrence of abuse were aggressive behaviors of the person with dementia and the caregiver's anxiety, depression, lower education, and higher perceived burden.

## Nursing Assessment of the Person With Dementia

The primary nursing responsibility related to elder abuse is to be on the alert for indicators of abuse and neglect when caring for people with dementia. It is important to recognize that elder abuse is usually well hidden, sometimes for a long time, and information may be purposefully withheld. Clues to elder abuse might first be noted when a vulnerable older person is seen in an emergency department or admitted to a hospital. Nurses may identify the indicators of elder abuse listed in Table 15.1 during a usual patient assessment, but when these conditions are identified, the pieces of the puzzle need to be put together to detect elder abuse or neglect.

======*FAST FACTS in a NUTSHELL*

It is imperative to be alert for indicators of elder abuse or neglect when assessing people who have dementia.

**CLINICAL SNAPSHOT:** When Mrs. P was admitted for a hip fracture, the nursing assessment noted that she had very poor hygiene, matted and oily hair, multiple bruises on her trunk and upper arms, and long toenails that curled under her toes. The nurse discussed this with Mrs. P's doctor and asked for further assessment of nutritional status and a referral for social services.

### TABLE 15.1  Nursing Assessment for Indicators of Elder Abuse or Neglect

| Assessment Parameter | What to Look for |
| --- | --- |
| Hydration | Dry mucous membranes, dry mouth, poor skin turgor over sternum and abdomen, concentrated urine |
| Nutrition | Dry, fissured, cracked lips; tongue and mucous membranes inflamed, ulcerated, or with white patches |
| Laboratory indicators for nutritional deficiency | Anemia; low serum glucose, sodium, potassium, ferritin, folate, or vitamin $B_{12}$; serum albumin level less than 5.5 g/dL; cholesterol levels less than 160 mg/dL; total iron-binding capacity less than 250 mcg/dL |
| Skin | Leg or pressure ulcers, poor wound healing |
| Injuries from falls, accidents, or abuse | Swelling; limited range of motion; evidence of burns from stoves, cigarettes, or hot water; marks from cuts, bites, or punctures |
| Bruise patterns characteristic of abuse | Bruises that reflect the shape of objects; bruises on the trunk, face, head, or both upper arms; bruises at various stages of healing (e.g., yellow, blue, red, purple) |
| Overall appearance | Weight loss, poor muscle tone, decreased strength, frailty, poor hygiene, edema, extremely long nails (including long toenails that interfere with mobility) |
| Indicators of excessive amounts of drugs or alcohol | Excessive somnolence, clouded mentation, slurred speech, staggering gait, difficulty walking, poor balance |
| Mood | Depressed, listless, apathetic, agitated |

## Nursing Assessment of Caregivers

In addition to assessing the person with dementia for the indicators listed in Table 15.1, nurses need to look for clues in the broader caregiver situation. For example, nurses have many opportunities to identify indicators of abuse or neglect in statements and actions of caregivers when they are visiting the person with dementia. Caregiving itself does not cause elder abuse; however, it can lead to abuse when those assuming the caregiving role are incapable of doing so because of life stresses, pathologic characteristics, personality characteristics, insufficient resources, or lack of understanding of the older adult's condition. Caregivers who perpetrate abuse often exhibit some of the same risk factors associated with abused elders, particularly if the caregivers themselves are older adults. Caregiver factors associated with elder abuse include poor health, cognitive impairment, social isolation, and dependence and co-residence, as well as poor interpersonal relations with the dependent elder. It is not unusual to have a mutually neglectful or abusive situation when an older married couple have several of the psychosocial risk factors just identified and are, in addition, socially isolated.

═══════════════════════════*FAST FACTS in a NUTSHELL*

A key indicator of elder abuse or neglect can be obtained through observation and documentation of caregivers.

**CLINICAL SNAPSHOT:** Mrs. E is in the cardiac intensive care unit with a diagnosis of myocardial infarction and she has a concomitant diagnosis of dementia. Upon admission, her personal appearance was unkempt and her blood tests indicate that she is malnourished. When her husband comes to visit, you note that his appearance is unkempt, his clothes are baggy, and he has trouble remembering and processing information. You request social service involvement for further assessment.

## Roles of Nurses

A primary role of nurses is to assess for indicators of abuse and to follow institutional policy for reporting suspected abuse to the public agency responsible for implementing adult protective service laws (as discussed in the next section). Nurses need to consider that adult protective service laws do not require reporters to *know* whether abuse or neglect has occurred, but merely to report it if they *suspect* its occurrence. The responsibility for problem verification rests with the public agency charged with implementing the law, not with the reporter or referral source. Nurses can find protocols and screening tools for elder mistreatment and abuse through the Internet sites listed in the Resources in a Nutshell section at the end of this chapter.

When elder abuse or neglect is caused by caregiver stress, nurses can initiate a referral for social services. Nurses also can incorporate the following interventions when they talk with care partners:

- Encourage families to reevaluate the demands of the situation and consider resources for support and assistance.
- Emphasize that care partners need to take care of themselves.
- Encourage care partners to find resources for delegating some of their responsibilities.
- Facilitate communication among all the decision makers, including the primary care provider, the older adult (if appropriate), and family members who are responsible for care.
- Suggest participation in educational or support groups.
- Identify patient's needs for skilled care and initiate referrals as appropriate (e.g., a recent fall may qualify the person for physical therapy or a change in medication may qualify the person for skilled nursing at home).
- Suggest types of medical equipment, disposable supplies, and assistive devices to improve function and safety for the elder and ease caregiver burden (e.g., caregivers may respond positively to suggestions about using grab bars for preventing falls in the bathroom).

## Adult Protective Service Laws

All states have adult protective services laws that address elder abuse and neglect. Although these laws differ, some common elements are pertinent to nurses:

- Reporting suspected abuse is mandatory in most states, and nurses are the health care workers most commonly identified as mandatory reporters.
- Most state laws protect the confidentiality of reports and the identity of all people involved in making them.
- Most reporting laws provide immunity for mandatory reporters, so nurses who act in good faith can report suspected cases without fear of liability.
- Penalties for failure to report include a charge of a misdemeanor, financial penalty, civil liability, or notification of the state licensing board.

## *FAST FACTS in a NUTSHELL*

It is important to become familiar with adult protective service laws that apply to a clinical practice setting and to follow protocols for reporting elder abuse and neglect.

## *RESOURCES in a NUTSHELL*

*Aging with Dignity*
*www.agingwithdignity.org*
- Information about advance directives

*Hartford Institute for Geriatric Nursing*
consultgerirn.org

- Decision Making and Dementia, *Try This,* Issue D9
- Elder Mistreatment and Abuse protocol
- Elder Mistreatment Assessment, *Try This,* Issue 15 and video illustrating application of the assessment tool

*National Center on Elder Abuse*

*www.ncea.aoa.gov*

*National Committee for the Prevention of Elder Abuse*

*preventelderabuse.org*

# 16

## Nursing Strategies to Address Caregiver Needs

### INTRODUCTION

*As discussed throughout this book, nurses who care for people with dementia address many dementia-related issues during the course of usual care. In addition to addressing the many ways in which dementia influences the daily care of your patients, you are likely to address the many ways in which this chronic condition affects your patients and their care partners over the long term. This may be especially evident when you develop a discharge plan and when family members and other care partners discuss their concerns with you. Although social workers are primarily responsible for addressing these needs, families of people with dementia often see nurses as a primary source of advice and guidance about dementia-related concerns. Thus, nurses are in key positions to teach about resources that address the needs of people with dementia and their care partners. This chapter provides an overview of types of resources that you need to be aware of so you can holistically address the dementia-related needs of your patients and their care partners as an integral part of your care plan.*

In this chapter, you will learn:

1. Relatively simple interventions to address caregiver needs
2. Information about respite care
3. Information about adult day centers
4. Information about care management services
5. Models of residential care for people with dementia
6. Information about hospice and palliative care for dementia

## NEEDS OF CAREGIVERS

Nurses who care for people with dementia are frequently aware of caregiver needs, which are likely to be exacerbated during times of hospitalization and other medical instabilities. The term "caregiver burden" describes the financial, physical, and psychosocial stresses that family members and other care partners experience during the course of dementia. Caregiver burden is associated with the following manifestations: depression; disturbed sleep; social isolation; job interruption; financial difficulties; lack of time for self; poor physical health; psychological, emotional, and mental strain; and feelings of anger, guilt, grief, anxiety, hopelessness, and helplessness. Nurses caring for people with dementia in short-term settings cannot address all the identified needs of caregivers; however, be aware of the manifestations of caregiver burden and express compassion. In addition, teach about the resources discussed in this chapter and encourage caregivers to participate in support and educational groups that address their concerns.

A relatively simple intervention is to teach about the Alzheimer's Association, which provides numerous resources that are available online and through local chapters everywhere in the United States. This resource can be "one-stop shopping" for information and referral through their 24/7 helpline at 800-272-3900. If the person resists your suggestion because of the word "Alzheimer's," you can emphasize that the association addresses needs of people with "related dementias" and "memory impairments" and is an excellent source of information for anyone dealing with similar issues. In addition, as part of the discharge plan, provide a copy of the Resources in a Nutshell section at the end of this chapter. This list includes information about all the types of resources that are commonly available for people with dementia and their care partners, as discussed in this chapter. When addressing issues specifically associated with mild, moderate, or advanced dementia, provide copies of the resource lists in Chapters 6 through 8.

## RESPITE CARE

Respite care refers to any service whose primary purpose is to relieve caregivers from their usual responsibilities for a short term. The typical recipient of respite care is a person with dementia who lives with a spouse, family member, or other care partner and requires daily or full-time assistance or supervision. Sources of respite care are:

- Adult day care
- Short-term care in a residential facility
- In-home companions or home health aides

Care partners can arrange for respite services when they need time off for work or for personal reasons—including stress reduction—or even for vacations. Nurses caring for people with dementia in acute care or other short-term care settings often are aware of the tremendous stress placed on care partners. In these situations, nurses can address the needs of the care partners by asking if they have considered using respite services and introduce this idea as a self-wellness intervention for the care partners. By initiating a discussion of respite care, you may be providing the "permission" that stressed caregivers need to take care of themselves.

===============*FAST FACTS in a NUTSHELL*

Nurses can suggest that caregivers consider respite services as a self-wellness intervention to reduce stress.

🌀 CLINICAL SNAPSHOT: Mr. U lives with his daughter and has been admitted for uncontrolled diabetes and hypertension. His daughter confides that she is feeling very stressed about being responsible for her father's care as his needs have increased significantly during the past 6 months. Her husband wants her to go with him for 5 days when he is attending a conference in a place they have always wanted to see. You tell her there are many options for short-term care for her father while she is gone and you make a referral for social services.

## ADULT DAY CENTERS

Adult day centers, which are available in most communities, provide structured activities in a group setting for older people with cognitive and functional impairments. Adult day centers typically provide meals, social and recreational activities, and one or more of the following services:

- Transportation
- Medication management
- Assistance with personal care
- Monitoring of health status
- Group outings
- Music and art activities
- Religious services

These programs usually are available on weekdays for up to 8 hours a day; less commonly, some services are available for longer hours and on weekends and holidays. Studies have confirmed that day care programs can improve quality of life for people with dementia as well as their care partners. For example, Zarit et al. (2011) found that adult day services improved behavior and sleep for participants with dementia and lowered their caregivers' exposure to stressors.

## CARE MANAGEMENT SERVICES

Because the needs of the person with dementia and their care partners change frequently, it is difficult to identify and arrange for the most appropriate services, which also change during the course of the condition. This becomes even more complex when the person with dementia has medical issues, which is the typical situation for nurses who work in health care settings. Another complicating factor is that the care partners may live out of town—or even out of the country—or may not be available for many other reasons. In some situations, there may not be any close family members or care partners to assist with implementing care plans following discharge. In all these situations, it may be helpful to contact a geriatric care manager who can serve as the primary care coordinator for the person with dementia. Care management roles and range of responsibilities include:

- Performing initial and on-going patient assessments
- Planning, implementing, and monitoring a comprehensive care plan
- Working closely with the person with dementia, their family members, support resources, and health care professionals to address the multifaceted needs

Care management services can be obtained through independent care managers or nonprofit or for-profit organizations, as listed in the Resources in a Nutshell section at the end of this chapter.

━━━━━━━━━━━━━━━━━━━━━━━━━*FAST FACTS in a NUTSHELL*

Available resources that can support caregivers include:

- Adult day centers, which are widely available, are beneficial for people with dementia and their care partners.
- Care management services are a resource for planning, implementing, and monitoring a care plan as the needs of the person with dementia and the needs of the person's care partners change.

## RESIDENTIAL FACILITIES

Although nurses usually are not involved with decisions about residential care for people with dementia, they are responsible for developing discharge plans that provide for safe and appropriate living arrangements. This is especially important when planning care for people with dementia who have medical conditions that require strict adherence to a treatment plan but do not meet the criteria for skilled care, as illustrated in the Clinical Snapshot at the end of this chapter. Also, because traditional nursing homes are often associated with negative images, nurses can encourage care partners to explore the newer models for residential care of people with dementia.

### Newer Models for Residential Care

Many nursing homes have developed *specialized dementia, or memory support, programs.* A typical dementia program in a nursing facility is a separate unit with controlled access and exit so the residents cannot leave without supervision. These programs are suitable for people with moderate-to-advanced dementia who have some degree of mobility and are able to participate in group activities. They are similar to other nursing home units in many ways, but the activities are developed specifically for people with dementia and all staff members are trained for dementia care.

Another recent development for residential care is a *dementia assisted living facility,* which is most appropriate for people with mild-to-moderate dementia. These facilities are either free standing or a part of a long-term care facility or continuing care community. Sometimes they are separate units with controlled access within a larger assisted living facility. A typical dementia assisted living facility is designed with 16 or more individual rooms in a square around a courtyard to permit residents safe access to the entire indoor and outdoor space. Shared space usually includes sitting rooms, a kitchen area, and large activity rooms. Residents participate in group activities, eat their meals in a dining room, and have assistance with activities of daily living.

*Small group homes,* which have been available for decades with varying levels of state and federal regulation, are another option for residential care of people with dementia. The Green House Project is a nonprofit organization that began in 2003 as an alternative to traditional nursing facilities and is approved for Medicare and Medicaid funds. These "small-house nursing homes" provide personalized care in intentional communities of 7–10 older adults with chronic conditions, including mild dementia. There were 99 Green House Project homes in 27 states in 2011, with the expectation that this project will continue to expand.

## HOSPICE AND PALLIATIVE CARE SERVICES

Hospice and palliative care services are increasingly available for people with dementia in any setting, but these programs are underutilized because of lack of awareness (Torke et al., 2010). The primary goal of hospice and palliative care programs is to provide support, comfort, and symptom management during the course of progressive illnesses such as dementia. Medicare and other health insurance programs cover both types of care, if certain requirements are met:

- A major difference is that eligibility for hospice requires that the person have a life expectancy of less than 6 months, and that recipients do not receive curative treatments.
- Palliative care services can be initiated for symptom management at any time during the course of dementia, but they generally are short-term.
- Palliative dementia care addresses issues such as the following: pain; loss of appetite; weakness; fatigue; anxiety; depression; sleep disturbances; behavioral changes; and social, emotional, psychological, and spiritual support to the individual and care partners.
- Hospice dementia care addresses these same issues as well as end-of-life concerns.

Nurses are in key positions to identify the need, teach about the benefits, and suggest that care partners explore options for these services. These services are appropriate for people with advanced dementia, even without other medical conditions, and for people with moderate dementia who also have other serious conditions. For example, people with advanced dementia may be admitted to the hospital for aspiration pneumonia because of dysphagia. These situations typically involve the placement of a nasogastric tube and a decision about long-term ways to provide nutrition. If a decision is made to forego a long-term feeding tube, hospice or palliative care services may be beneficial for assisting with comfort feeding and other related issues. Refer to Chapters 8 and 15 for information about palliative care and decisions related to care of people with advanced dementia.

## ═══════════════════════════════*FAST FACTS in a NUTSHELL*

A wide range of new residential models, along with hospice and palliative care services, addresses dementia-related issues and provide social, emotional, psychological, and spiritual support to people with dementia and their care partners.

### 🔆 CLINICAL SNAPSHOT: DISCHARGE PLANS FOR A PATIENT WITH CONGESTIVE HEART FAILURE

During the past 6 months, Sophie Walker has been admitted three times to the medical floor where you work for exacerbation of congestive heart failure. After the first admission, she received care in a skilled nursing facility for 10 days and then insisted on returning to her own home to manage her care independently. When Sophie's condition worsened after a month, she was readmitted to the hospital and then discharged to home after 3 days. She qualified for skilled nursing services from the visiting nurse association and remained stable for 2 months. When she was admitted the third time, she had not been taking her medications correctly and the mental status assessment indicated progressive memory impairment and other cognitive limitations. Because she attended social and nutrition programs at the local senior center, she was not homebound and no longer qualified for skilled nursing services to assist with her medical management at home. Sophie's doctor indicated that the repeated hospitalizations could be prevented if her medications were managed appropriately and her medical condition monitored closely. When Sophie's daughter visits, she confides that she is very frustrated because she is the only family member involved with her mother's care and she lives 300 miles away and works full time. You give her the list of the Resources in a Nutshell

*(continued)*

*(continued)*

from this chapter and suggest she contact a geriatric care manager to assist her with developing a plan. You also provide information about dementia assisted living facilities and suggest she explore options with her mother.

## ═══════════════RESOURCES in a NUTSHELL

### Alzheimer's Association

*www.alz.org*

- "One-stop shopping" for information about support and education groups and all resources discussed in this chapter
- 24/7 helpline for advice and information about all types of resources: 800-272-3900

### Family Caregiver Alliance

*www.caregiver.org*

- Information about dementia, stresses of caregiving, and resources for family caregivers

### Green House Project

*www.thegreenhouseproject.org*

- Information about Green House Project homes

### Helpguide

*www.helpguide.org*

- Information about dementia and caregiver issues
- Links to resources, including respite, adult day care, and hospice and palliative care

### National Association of Professional Geriatric Care Managers

*www.caremanager.org*

- Information about geriatric care managers
- Directory of geriatric care managers by zip codes

### National Eldercare Locator

*eldercare.gov*

- Information specialists available Monday to Friday 9 a.m. to 8 p.m. ET at 800-677-1116 or online

### National Hospice and Palliative Care Organization

*www.nhpco.org*

- Information about hospice and palliative care for dementia

# References

Alzheimer's Association. (2009, January). *Characteristics, costs and health service use for Medicare beneficiaries with a dementia diagnosis.* Washington, DC: Author.

Alzheimer's Society. (2008). *Dementia: Out of the shadows.* London, UK: Author.

Alzheimer's Society. (2010). *My name is not dementia: People with dementia discuss quality of life.* London, UK: Author.

American Geriatrics Society Panel on the Pharmacologic Management of Persistent Pain in Older Persons. (2009). Pharmacologic management of persistent pain in older persons. *Journal of the American Geriatrics Society, 57,* 1331–1346.

Arrighi, H. M., Neumann, P. J., Lieberburg, I. M., & Townsend, R. J. (2010). Lethality of Alzheimer's disease and its impact on nursing home placement. *Alzheimer Disease and Associated Disorders, 24*(1), 90–95.

Banerjee, S. (2009). *The use of antipsychotic medication for people with dementia: Time for action.* Retrieved from UK Department of Health website: http://www.dh.gov.uk/en/Publicationsandstatistics/Publications/PublicationsPolicyAndGuidance/DH_108303

Goin, L., Duke, L., Hollawell, D., Horton, A., & Voytek, M. W. (2011). Ambulation and mobility. In G. A. Martin & M. N. Sabbagh (Eds.), *Palliative care for advanced Alzheimer's and dementia* (pp. 131–151). New York, NY: Springer Publishing Company.

Husebo, B. S., Ballard, C., Sandvik, R., Nilsen, O. B., & Aarsland, D. (2011). Efficacy of treating pain to reduce behavioural disturbances in residents of nursing homes with dementia: Cluster randomised clinical trial. *British Medical Journal, 343,* d4065.

Huybrechts, K. F., Rothman, K. J., Siliman, R. A., Brookhart, M. A., & Schneeweiss, S. (2011). Risk of death and hospital admission for major medical events after initiation of psychotropic medications in older adults admitted to nursing homes. *Canadian Medical Association Journal, 183*(7), E411–E419.

Inouye, S., van Dyck, C., Alessi, C. A., Balkin, S., Diegal, A., & Horwitz, R. (1990). Clarifying confusion: The confusion assessment method. *Annals of Internal Medicine, 113*(12), 941–948.

LaReau, R., Benson, L., Watcharotone, K., & Manguba, G. (2008). Examining the feasibility of implementing specific nursing interventions to promote sleep. *Geriatric Nursing, 29*(3), 197–206.

Legler, A., Bradley, E. H., & Carlson, M. D. A. (2011). The effect of comorbidity burden on health care utilization for patients with cancer using hospice. *Journal of Palliative Medicine, 14*(6), 751–756.

Maher, A. R., Maglione, M., Bagley, S., Suttorp, M., Hu, J.-H., Ewing, B., . . . Shekelle, P. G. (2011). Efficacy and comparative effectiveness of atypical antipsychotic medications for off-label uses in adults: A systematic review and meta-analysis. *Journal of the American Medical Association, 306*(12), 1359–1369.

Maslow, K. (2006). How many people with dementia are hospitalized? In N. M. Silverstein & K. Maslow (Eds.), *Improving hospital care for persons with dementia* (pp. 3–21). New York, NY: Springer Publishing Company.

McKhann, G. M., Knopman, D. S., Chertkow, H., Hyman, B. T., Jack, C. R., Kawas, C. H., . . . Phelps, C. H. (2011). The diagnosis of dementia due to Alzheimer's disease: Recommendations from the National Institute on Aging-Alzheimer's Association workgroups on diagnostic guidelines for Alzheimer's disease. *Alzheimer's & Dementia, 7*(3), 263–269.

National Hospice and Palliative Care Organization. (2010, September). *NHPCO facts and figures: Hospice care in America.* Alexandria, VA: Author.

Power, G. A. (2010). I want to go home. In G. A. Power (Ed.), *Dementia beyond drugs: Changing the culture of care* (pp. 191–213). Baltimore, MD: Health Professions Press.

Reisberg, B. (1986). Dementia: A systematic approach to identifying reversible causes. *Geriatrics, 41*(4), 30–46.

Rudolph, J. L., Zanin, N. M., Jones, R. M., Marcantonio, E. R., Fong, T. G., Uang, F. M., & Inouye, S. K. (2010). Hospitalization in community-dwelling persons with Alzheimer's disease: Frequency and causes. *Journal of the American Geriatrics Society, 58*(8), 1542–1548.

Sabbagh, M. N., McCarthy, M., & Martin, G. A. (2011). Determining and defining advanced dementia. In G. A. Martin & M. N. Sabbagh (Eds.), *Palliative care for advanced Alzheimer's and dementia* (pp. 3–9). New York, NY: Springer Publishing Company.

Snyder, L. (2010). *Living your best with early-stage Alzheimer's.* North Branch, MN: Sunrise River Press.

Torke, A. M., Holtz, L. R., Hui, S., Castelluccio, P., Connor, S., Eaton, M. A., . . . Sachs, G. A. (2010). Palliative care for patients with dementia: A national survey. *Journal of the American Geriatrics Society, 58*(11), 2114–2121.

U.S. Preventive Services Task Force. (2009). Screening for depression in adults: U.S. Preventive Services Task Force recommendation statement. *Annals of Internal Medicine, 151,* 784–792.

Van der Steen, J. T. (2010). Dying with dementia: What we know after more than a decade of research. *Journal of Alzheimer's Disease, 22,* 37–55.

Wiglesworth, A., Mosqueda, L., Mulnard, R., Liao, S., Gibbs, L., & Fitzgerald, W. (2010). Screening for abuse and neglect of people with dementia. *Journal of the American Geriatrics Society, 58,* 493–500.

Wollen, K. A. (2010). Alzheimer's disease: The pros and cons of pharmaceutical, nutritional, botanical, and stimulatory therapies, with a discussion of treatment strategies from the perspective of patients and practitioners. *Alternative Medicine Review, 15*(3), 223–244.

Zarit, S. H., Kim, K., Femia, E. E., Almeida, D. M., Savia, J., & Molenaar, P. C. (2011). Effects of adult day care on daily stress of caregivers: A within-person approach. *Journals of Gerontology, Series B: Psychology Sciences and Social Sciences, 66B*(5), 538–546. doi:10.1093/geronb/gbr030

# Index

Printed in the United States
By Bookmasters